INJUSTICE AND PROPHECY IN THE AGE OF MASS INCARCERATION

The Politics of Sanity

Andrew Skotnicki

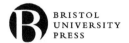

BRISTOL
UNIVERSITY
PRESS

First published in Great Britain in 2022 by

Bristol University Press
University of Bristol
1–9 Old Park Hill
Bristol
BS2 8BB
UK
t: +44 (0)117 374 6645
e: bup-info@bristol.ac.uk

Details of international sales and distribution partners are available at bristoluniversitypress.co.uk

British Library Cataloguing in Publication Data
A catalogue record for this book is available from the British Library

ISBN 978-1-5292-2221-0 hardcover
ISBN 978-1-5292-2223-4 ePub
ISBN 978-1-5292-2224-1 ePdf

Cover design: Liam Roberts
Front cover image: coldsnowstorm/iStock
Bristol University Press use environmentally responsible print partners.
Printed in Great Britain by CPI Group (UK) Ltd, Croydon, CR0 4YY

Contents

Introduction

There is a social psychological and, often, personal sense of dismay, trepidation, and irritation among the general population when confronted by persons of low status with acute psychological distress or by those with a radical political message. At the same time, detention facilities in nations such as Great Britain and the United States are more and more filled with representatives of these populations.

The pathos and seeming hopelessness of their plight is poignantly captured by George Orwell in the character of the unwitting and helpless revolutionary, Winston, in the novel, *1984*. Under torture by the effortlessly composed bureaucrat, O'Brien, Winston is reminded by his tormentor of the cost of resistance to the "sane" directives of the State: "You would not make an act of submission which is the price of sanity. You preferred to be a lunatic."[1]

Allow me to share a vignette that captures the ubiquitous reality of "lunatics" in penal institutions here and abroad. In the several dozen university classes on the theological and ethical implications of the criminal justice system that I have taught to confined men and women in the jails of New York City and one of its neighboring counties, I always attempt to give the students who accompany me from our main campus an impactful experience on who goes to jail and who does not. One common exercise is to ask the incarcerated students how many in their housing units are either on psychotropic medications or show demonstrative signs of acute psychological and emotional distress. The impact of the instantaneous responses is more visceral than simply numerical: there are forced exhales, eyebrows instinctively raise, heads begin to shake; all affirming that the numbers are striking. The dramatic emphasis of the reactions unfailingly shocks and disturbs the visitors far more than the simple reporting of statistical evidence.[2]

The inevitable question raised by the preceding experience among my students and, hopefully, the reader—hinted at in the Orwell quote—is part of what I wish to explore in this volume: Why do we punish so many of those determined to be mentally ill? Suffice to say for now that the data fully confirm that the anecdote just related accurately portrays their overwhelming numbers among the incarcerated population.

The other task of the book is to investigate a premise; one that is far less glaring but of the utmost importance; and it will be my intention to explore its multiple dimensions in detail. I will contend that there is something about those determined to be insane (especially those who are poor and disenfranchised), those out of step cognitively and emotionally with established norms of intelligence and moral perception, that evokes the instinctive denunciation among those considered to be normal to which we have alluded. This stance, translated into structural policy, is intensified by a virtual monopoly on the part of the therapeutic/psychiatric community in providing largely irrefutable scientific documentation of the unsuitability of many of our fellow citizens to live in consort with the rest of us. It is further compounded by a Social Darwinist/neoliberal ideology of free market largesse complemented by an aggravated emphasis on personal responsibility for the ills, anger, or, even, the aggravated eccentricities of those who dwell outside the domain of the comfortable and well-to-do.

To reframe the question and premise: just as crime is a social creation so too is cerebral malfunction.[3] That is not to say, in reference to writers like Thomas Szasz, that the latter is an elaborate fabrication, but it is to say that the political economy/mental illness dyad is very much in play and will be a significant focus of the argument in the pages to come.[4] By way of comparison, it is illustrative, if not deeply ironic, that the various logical and expressive maladies of the privileged (including, quite possibly, some of my university students) bear little or no social stigma, are invariably treated in private psychiatric or therapeutic consultations, in online or in-person support groups, or in the comforts of the home, whereas a large segment of those determined to have abject behavioral deficiencies, or who supplement those presumed deficiencies with a publicly proclaimed political vision wildly out of step with the prevailing social compact, are herded into forced confinement.[5]

While I will investigate a series of explanations for this phenomenon, the one that will emerge most consistently is the relation between "insanity" and prophecy. There is, in other words, something in the message or insight that certain unconventional people convey that is an outrage to the socioeconomic and cultural consensus and to the uneasy psychological, emotional, and spiritual stability of the "sane" population. The oracles of the unwanted coincide with the traditional role of what Max Weber calls the emissary prophet, whose communication, spoken or merely theatrical, is to critique and discomfort any established order that aggrandizes the rich and comfortable at the expense of those too destitute or weak to mount significant protest and, even more poignantly, fulfil the gift and promise of a fully human life.[6]

The concept of prophecy, like all theological constructs, is a rich and varied one so it behooves us from the start to make clear the notion of the emissary to which we have just alluded. Many of the religions of the ancient Near East had prophets or prophetic castes who were attached to the court, ruler, or potentate and served both a ceremonial role as well as an intercessory and magical one vis-à-vis the forces of the cosmos. In its early manifestations, this was the case of prophecy in Israel.[7] Such court functionaries were legitimized by virtue of the power of the office itself and directed their revelatory utterances to the king or queen rather than to the people at large. At the same time, they were subject to constraints by the very security bestowed upon them by the monarch, thus, by definition, compromising the illimitable transcendence of the divine and the often-inscrutable messages they were commanded to proffer.[8]

The prophets with whom we will be concerned, in Michael Walzer's terminology, are not of the court or temple but of the "street." They are lone individuals touched by a compelling intuition or actual revelation of appointment from a transcendent, overpowering, and empirically opaque source. They, as those who preceded them, possess no authority accruing to their social, political, or religious standing; whatever influence they may exert is the direct result of the effect their actions or oracles might summon from the society and its ruling elites whose actions prompted the deity to instill their "fiercely antipolitical radicalism."[9]

This radicalism on behalf of the voiceless and powerless also distinguishes to a significant degree these prophets from the vibrant culture of confrontation, with its frequent religious denunciations of moral waywardness, if not diabolical corruption, that so strongly characterizes contemporary political discourse in America and elsewhere. Cathleen Kaveny has traced the evolution of the American "jeremiad" (a linguistic play on the name of the prophet, Jeremiah) both in its biblically based covenantal origins in the nascent Puritan community in Massachusetts, as well as in its later manifestations on behalf of natural rights and/or the ethical substance of a given party's governing platform.[10]

Here, prophecy tends to serve in each instance, however distinct, an American messianism wherein policies are evaluated against a parochial national horizon and, often, personal or group self-interest. By way of contrast, the perspective offered by this volume's catalogue of prophets is, at best, peripheral to the credo of American exceptionalism with its inevitable emphases on economic growth, national security, and the periodic demonstration of mass violence. More to the point, these messengers are, to a person, outcasts, not political players.[11]

Nor is our exposition to be likened to the popular conception of the prophet as one attuned in some prescient way to future events and, commonly, apocalyptic events. One might think here of doomsday cults and the welter of gnostic and Manichean mediums predicting the violent end of history, normally with self-righteous and almost gleeful anticipation.[12]

We will have much more to say about the prophets about whom we will speak but one thing will be abundantly clear: such witnesses are always persecuted and, as history unfailingly reveals, branded as lunatics, dangers to society, irrational to the point of incoherence, and duly punished for it. That is to say, unlike other incarnations of the social critic possessed by a perceived otherworldly warrant, *all* of those heard from or referred to in our study have felt the exclusion and violence of life in jail or prison. Furthermore, they, like the schizophrenics, and, not uncommonly, obdurate political radicals, are normally ensconced in pockets of urban poverty and racial prejudice; inhabitants of a world that mocks the regnant materialist epistemology, its facile, computational, and ultimately hierarchical measure of human worth, and its accompanying normative and punitive constraints.

I will build the argument—one that Karl Jaspers perceptively acknowledged—that to dwell in this mysterious realm often involves a deep religious experience as opposed to what is commonly denoted as some perverted psychological or psychopathological condition.[13] For these clairvoyants receive an instinctive summons from a whole far greater than the parts constituted by external sensation. And, true to the long-standing determination of medical and therapeutic experts, suffer a mental malady precisely because many receive "visions" or hear "voices"—a condition one psychiatric scholar identifies as a "grossly misleading" "delusion."[14] Furthermore, that mysterious and unsettling voice always invades the prophetic heart to speak and act on behalf of those too frail to plead their own cause. As Abraham Heschel observes, the primary prophetic activity is "*interference*." It involves demands that those so chosen, or, in many cases, so afflicted, remonstrate about wrongs imposed upon others, that they meddle in affairs which are seemingly neither their concern nor their responsibility.[15]

Such a "calling" has always brought recrimination, minimally, and most tellingly, condemnation, banishment, incarceration, and not infrequently, loss of life. It is thus far from hyperbolic to recall Andrew Scull's contention that to be judged insane, particularly in countries such as America and England, makes one prone to endure "a kind of social, mental, and metaphysical death."[16] In line with our guiding premise, the "mad," particularly since the advent of capitalist economies and the Age of Reason, have posed both a symbolic and practical threat to the very fabric of civil society, specifically due to the disjunction between the canons of reasonable discourse, that is, common sense, and the ravings and uncanny histrionics born in the secret domain of the imagination. Scull notes correctly that those deemed to be feeble-minded are, in reality, unbearably troublesome and constitute by their "looming presence" a "source of profound stress on the lives of those forced to cope with them." We may revile them, laugh at them, or simply turn up our noses and pass by but "in the shadows lurks a darker perspective, from which they are viewed as an explosive mix of menace and misery."[17]

Our study is not a history per se, although a topic as varied and complex as rational inadaptability cannot be adequately grasped without an understanding, indeed appreciation, for the ways in which unconventional demeanor has been viewed and treated over a wide chronological continuum. This is particularly relevant also given a hermeneutic based upon the prophetic vocation. It is this interpretive lens that I believe provides an essential insight into the penchant and, given the social and psychological lacunae of "sane" population—about which I will argue in detail—the need to sequester and punish those working within exceptional (writ irrational) imaginative frameworks.

I will orchestrate the theme that what distinguishes how many of those deemed insane are treated now as opposed to the way their condition was addressed in ages past is not, remembering Henri Bergson, a difference in degree but in kind.[18] Put simply, our pre-modern ancestors were not particularly more magnanimous in the face of eccentric individuals, but the substance of their reaction was determined by what the incomprehensible behavior of these persons revealed about who they are: people touched by or, perhaps, possessed by forces and powers that commanded wariness, fear, and awe, a species of the *tremendum et fascinans* of which Rudolf Otto speaks.[19] On the other hand, I will insist that the profound disquiet the mad currently evoke, a disquiet that rouses those of us in the normal majority to silence them and shutter them *en masse* in penal facilities, is explicable not due to who *they* but due to who *we* are. They hold up a mirror that challenges any smug assurance of normalcy and moral rectitude and, more to the point, any pretense to social, psychological, and spiritual well-being. Their message is intolerable on a number of levels, many of them nestled in remote corners of the psyche, but not a whit less serious in their consequence for the uneasy state of mind of the man or woman on the street, or for the displaced throng who trouble them, shut away in the jails and prisons of our land.

The study will require a nuanced appreciation, with no small amount of censure, of the role of the therapeutic and psychiatric professions. As stated, the history of both is complex and, like all disciplines, each has its catalogue of heroes and villains. That said, the latter is not my predominant concern. The critique presented here is broader and more focused on metaethical concerns rather than discrete actions by individuals and associations in a specific temporal sequence. For it is the language that is used to describe those perceived as "dimwitted," again heavily tilted toward racial minorities and the poor, that troubles me, a language that all but determines the social, therapeutic, legal, and, more often than not, penal response that relegates those so labeled as unfit to live among us. We will explore the moral parameters of that discourse and highlight the narrow list of alternatives the designation of insanity leaves to health-care professionals, the police, the courts, and society at large, remembering that the ominous specter of madness has laid the groundwork for those dismissive and aggressive responses.

In short, I am investigating how our culture responds to those with dissonant and disruptive cognitive and emotional frameworks. As Amanda Pustilnik writes, the "lock-ups" to which those coined as crazy are consigned are but a projection of the "prisons of the mind" that ensnare us personally and as a society. We are, as she writes, "trapped in our thoughts about them" and the only way to end the injustice of branding and banishing those that pierce us so deeply is "to think them out first."[20] That will not be an easy task given the issues that we will discuss in the following pages. For our intolerance follows the predictable path, trodden repeatedly over the centuries, that maniacal intuitions often bear a haunting echo of the message of the prophets who preceded them. Whether their forced exile will come to an end and their human dignity be restored depends in large part upon whether we can acknowledge our fears and the social structural constraints that keep these contemporary prophets at a safe distance from our sight but hardly far from our anxious state of mind.

The first chapter will address a series of issues essential to the analytical task of probing the mental illness/jailhouse betrothal. It will first trace the radically disparate ways the phenomenon of insanity has been understood over the course of time, discussing biblical, classical, and other pre-modern arrangements with "psychosis" before turning its attention to the decisive shift to forcible institutionalization beginning with the transition to capitalist economies after the demise of feudalism and the rise of mercantilism; a paradigmatic shift that reached its peak in the mid-eighteenth century. It will also provide a similar brief overview of the history of psychiatry since the changes within that discipline have moved through similar alteration, not only regarding the legitimacy of metaphysical inspiration, but also in the diminution of Freudian, Jungian, and other methodologies respectful of the role of the unconscious. In their place, there has been a marked emphasis on a strictly materialist, biological rendering of questionable cerebral functioning, accompanied by a virtual monopoly of medical and juridical discretion in deciding who is and who is not capable of functioning outside the barbed wire confines of the local detention facility.

Chapter 2 will explore theological and philosophical sources that account for the massive shift in worldviews that normalized two disparate strategies in response to the ravings of the "mad" and the foibles of the "sane." Nietzsche and Foucault are particularly helpful in this task as they underscore the shattering of a largely wholistic, non-binary reaction to those floundering in the cognitive mainstream that characterized the traditional approach with "a moral genealogy" predicated upon the unimpeachable authority of those who have elevated themselves to a role of political and economic superiority. It is at this juncture that the concept of "man," in Nietzschean parlance, was first brought into being, a creature definitively categorized by measurable performance in accord with heavily constrictive statutory and bureaucratic constraints. The discussion will blend with the suppositions of philosophical and perceptual dualism that furnish the necessary intellectual and moral stance for the guiltless desire to omit realms of experience, and classes of people, who fall outside the hyper-comparative and evaluative perspective part and parcel of a binary vision of the world.

The third chapter will analyze why those considered to be mentally ill are so often punished. Socioeconomic, psychological, and theological factors will be considered. As to the first, the neoliberal fusion of an unfettered free market paired with an invasive scrutiny of individual conduct on the part of the law enforcement and security industries has played a substantial role in the massive rise in penal commitments in countries such as the United States and England over the last half century. The rudiments of neoliberal philosophy coincide with what Loic Wacquant calls a "hyperincarceration" pattern: the disproportionate attention to and detention of citizens predicated not upon the proscribed action as such, but upon their class, race, and geographical location.[21] This strategy is brought into sharper focus by a high concentration of arrests of those lacking political clout for "nuisance crimes."[22] A recent study reported that of the 800 people who spent the most time revolving in and out of the jail system in New York City, over half were homeless. The charges for which they were arrested in these cases were petit larceny, drug possession, and trespassing.[23] If one adds to this the dearth of public facilities for those categorized as mentally ill, it becomes a short ride to institutionalization, not in an ambulance, but in a police van.

The psychological section, with distinct theological overtones, will work mainly with the ideas of Kierkegaard on the pervasive depression that all experience due to the human dichotomy between an unlimited imagination and a progressively limited physicality. Kierkegaard argues that it is those who honestly face this psychological morass who often devolve into fantasy and, at least seeming, fabrication (the profile of most schizophrenics), while the "sane" majority tend to lose themselves in denial and identification with the prevailing cultural and moral status quo. I will contend that the mad bedevil the majority and remind them of their alienation from their true condition; the latter then employ what Rene Girard calls the "scapegoat mechanism" to silence and quarantine those whose presence is a troubling token of the depths of their inner disquiet.[24]

Finally, continuing the spiritual motif begun with Kierkegaard, I will discuss the ineffability of religious experience, using the work of William James among many others, and the limited moral language that overdetermines a persistent diagnosis of psychosis and a-sociability for persons who have "out of body" experiences, hear voices, or have corporeal visions.

In the fourth chapter, we will provide a characterological depiction of the "mad" prophet. Basically, the prophet announces or conveys a message that virtually no one wants to hear, most of all those whose material and psychological profiles are held up to withering and, in my opinion, indefensible scrutiny by the unwanted and disturbing presence of those seen as psychologically and socially incompetent. Among the issues that we will discuss, two are most pertinent to the book's argument: common sense and insight. The relation between the two will be examined in detail but, briefly, just as paradigms in science condition and limit all investigation in accord with the ongoing and seemingly unassailable foundational dogma, so the canons of common sense provide not only epistemological comfort but also strictly dismiss and limit ideas that upset the smooth functioning of mental processes and the operative conventional wisdom. In contrast, insight is always meddlesome, irksome, and, often, prophetic, since, by definition, it challenges the inherent conservatism of what is commonly held to be true, even if its determinations result in the debasement of those whose presence and message challenge such ready-at-hand conclusions.

Chapter 5 will explore the question of who, exactly, are the contemporary prophets. Here, I will embellish a distinction that will be referred to often in the text: that between involuntary and voluntary prophets. The former assemblage is constituted by those whose life condition, invariably mired in poverty and social immobility, invokes spontaneous feelings of acute distress, frequently accompanied by the wild comportment and adverse reaction toward the citizenry at large that has led to their seizure and forcible removal from public spaces. In effect, their unconventional conduct is at least partially spurred by their eviscerated social forecast that provokes an instinctive rage against the civic order and the forces allayed against the development of their human potential and that of those for whom they care. Thus, the "angry young man" or woman, or the ragged and displaced with their frequently incomprehensible ravings, should not simply be reduced to the status of the incorrigible, or even socio-pathological, but serve as a gnawing reminder of the daily horrors confronted by so many in general, and by the urban poor in particular. This is not to dismiss the obligation all have to respect the lives and goods of others, but to add a challenging hermeneutical element to the legal and especially penal response that unlawful or disquieting actions inevitably provoke.

This exposition will be followed by a profile of the voluntary prophet, one who has the conviction that he or she has been chosen by God, or by some unseen and, normally, unsought herald, to deliver an urgent message. That missive is always explosive in its substance as well as its intent. It seeks to undermine definitively any social, political, and economic structure that debases the sacredness of creature and creation. It is always a fervent and impatient cry on behalf of the downtrodden, and it is forcibly silenced to the degree that those instrumental in operating the machinery of production and the arrest and detention of the deviant have felt its message pierce their levels of comfort and self-satisfaction. We will discuss the difficulties inherent in the prophetic vocation, not the least of which is a persistent sense of loneliness, alienation, and affliction—the very psychological factors so often identified with those who succumb to psychosis.

In reference to both prophetic types, I will orchestrate the narrative with examples and quotes from those who have and continue to bear the weight of such a perilous stance in a world obsessed with security and comfort, often at almost any price. The chapter will end with a brief exposition on the prison as the sanctuary of the prophets. If all that is written in this book has explanatory merit, then the prison is far from the domain of the misanthrope; it is, in a progressively advanced manner, the dwelling place of those whose message most of us cannot and will not tolerate. Mental illness is the *crime de jour* that justifies the muting of the prophetic voice.

It is important for the argument being presented to add a brief linguistic note at this juncture. The reader will often see the words *sane* and *insane* in quotation marks. This show of irony is meant to underline the insidious way that labels with no consistent empirical and theoretical foundation, save the rigid boundaries between those who do and do not fit into an acquisitive, status-driven, and exclusionary culture, serve to nourish pre-reflexive judgments on the human and social worth of the maligned cohort about whom we will speak.

If, as Louis Sass attests, "the madman is a protean figure in the Western imagination," then, among his many façades, surely the prophet is an apt descriptor given the panorama of responses to uncommon demeanor that we will consider in the pages to come.[25]

It is the nature of theology, not just prophecy, to offer alternatives (insights) to any entrenched order that lacks a historical appreciation for the role of grace and providence and, remembering Hegel, the "cunning" restlessness that must never derive satisfaction from the current state of affairs, especially when so many have grown diffident, or simply apathetic, to the daily specter of the swelling numbers wallowing in the gutter.

Despite the historical and social contractarian factors that have largely narrowed the domain of the theological discipline to the ivory tower or the pulpit, any reticence regarding a public stance in this matter can no longer be justified. There are far too many who have suffered and are suffering after having been professionally diagnosed as being out of their minds, summarily dismissed, and carted away to bastions of secrecy, violence, and dehumanization. This is hardly an issue of religious meddling in the secular; it is an issue of human dignity. There is no faith or doctrinal requirement attached to the insistence that each human being is an end in herself, and that many are susceptible to interior impulses and motivations that often transcend not only the constraints of the empirical but also shed new and creative light on established patterns of thought and social interaction.

The fact, as our title suggests, that the subjugation of a vast assembly, both implicitly and explicitly, to maintain the privilege and comfort of those self-defined as lucid often summons insights from the former, who are then branded as deranged and duly castigated, does not diminish the authenticity of the insight nor the vocation of the one who proffers it. As Leo Strauss reminds us, in a world where spiritual matters are subjected to and often dominated by "ratio," it is the office of theology "to bring to life for our era 'the irrational in the idea of the Divine.'"[26]

This book will seek to honor the world's most dangerous profession and, at the same time, prod the conscience of those of us who think we are healthy because we are surrounded by companions mired in the same failed attempt to circumvent both personal and social self-deception.

Overview of the Problem of Mental Illness and Incarceration

We begin our investigation with sociological and historical data that underscore the evolution of mental illness from a local and, for the most part, equivocal reaction to human eccentricity, one never far from holy fear, if not cautious respect, to the current pervasiveness of faulting and punishing many people who, putatively, have no control over the condition that does so much to define them. We will look at the numbers to get a statistical appreciation of the depth of the problem, trace the evolution of the way the phenomenon has been addressed historically, and detail the authoritative rise of medical diagnoses as fully determinative of the psychopathic condition and the shrunken alternatives, save incarceration, available for those so diagnosed. In complementary fashion, we will also discuss the growing dissatisfaction within the psychiatric community with a, largely, Freudian and Jungian emphasis on the integrity of the unconscious and the methods there prescribed to appreciate and illumine the determinative power of inner forces, as distinct from the current emphasis on strictly biological explanations for uncanny and unacceptable behavior.

Statistical data

If anything, a pragmatic, writ positivist, public ideology, especially in an age of dwindling social services and increased revenue opportunities for the corporate and financial sectors, would easily surmise that it is far more cost-effective to treat a person designated as psychotic in an out-patient or in-patient treatment context, or in a therapeutically centered mental health court, than foot the bill for an often-lengthy stay in a penal institution.[1]

The 2018–19 annual report of HM Prison & Probation Service revealed a cost of £41,136 per prisoner in the UK.[2] In America, the Vera Institute of Justice discloses that in a 40-state survey, representing more than 1.2 million confined persons, the annual individual cost averaged $31,286 and ranged from $14,603 in Kentucky to $60,076 in New York.[3] The latter number is particularly noteworthy since the three largest concentrations of the "mentally ill" in the US are not in health-care facilities but penal institutions; all of which are located in large urban centers with a comparatively high cost of living: the Los Angeles County Jail, the Cook County Jail in Chicago, and the Rikers Island jail complex in New York City.[4] In fact, the New York City Comptroller, in a 2018 report, revealed that the municipal correctional budget, when divided by the total number of the incarcerated, amounted to $302,296 per person.[5]

As noted, we will delve in detail into what I perceive to be the reasons for this counterintuitive, dare I say liberal, financial extravagance. But it is beyond refute that one area of social policy—forcible detention of certain categories of the population, especially those with a medical or juridical prognosis of insanity—has, for the most part, escaped the sharp chisel of the fiscal sculptors.[6]

When one looks at the staggering number of those branded as disordered, psychotic, or schizophrenic in the cell blocks of our jails and prisons the lesson for our purposes is as clear as the closing numbers of the British Stock Exchange or the Dow on Wall Street. Of the 85,000 persons imprisoned in England and Wales in 2017, it is estimated that 90% suffer from "mental health issues" and approximately one-half show symptoms of depression and anxiety.[7] In its last comprehensive report on the matter, the Bureau of Justice Statistics (US Department of Justice) related that "more than half of all prison and jail inmates had a mental health problem." This included "705,600 inmates in State prisons, 78,800 in Federal prisons, and 479,900 in local jails. These estimates represent 56% of State prisoners, 45% of Federal prisoners, and 64% of jail inmates."[8] In the words of Pustilnik: "It is beyond cavil that the criminal justice system functions as the United States' [and by extension, Britain's] default asylum system."[9] Furthermore, statistics reveal the disturbing fact that between 30 and 40 percent of mentally ill individuals in the jails of certain states had no criminal charges whatsoever pending against them.[10]

There are larger political, economic, and cultural issues involved than these numerical snapshots reveal but it is certain that an authoritative diagnosis of cerebral malfunction for those whose condition is shrouded in the threat, if not the expression, of deviance, habitually culminates with its bearer behind bars.

The reader may be familiar with the extensive shuttering of the once ubiquitous public health facilities in the United States and Great Britain. The number of psychiatric beds in England numbered 152,000 in 1954; two decades later, the total had been reduced to 43,000.[11] In America, in 1955, state-run facilities housed 559,000 persons; by 2006 the number had shrunk to 49,000.[12] Those hundreds of thousands of souls have been augmented by the whopping numbers of the jail-bound, many of them out of step in the sanity parade, who have been summarily flushed into the tanks of the penal complex as the refuse of the great incarceration boom of the last half century.[13] To make matters even worse, on average, they serve, depending on the source, sentences from five to 12 months longer than other detainees for the same categories of offense.[14] Clearly, those aggregated within the "at risk" algorithm provoke personal and structural responses far more retaliatory and disturbing than those proceeding from practical political and monetary calculation. The masses of those labeled as psychotics in our "correctional" centers, literally in harm's way, preyed upon in multiple ways by both the confined population and, at least indirectly, by the silent complicity and ennui of staff and administrators, have been swept from our streets but not our psyche.[15] They do indeed haunt the collective and individual conscience in ways few of us understand. Before we delve into the dimensions of why we punish people determined to have a cognitive disability, it is crucial for our study to remember that the shame and opprobrium that surround this population have not been their consistent historical companions. Indeed, they were once, like Hermes, the messengers of the gods.

The ever-shifting understanding of madness

Biblical and pre-modern sources

St. Paul (I Cor. 14:1–2) writes: "Follow the way of love and eagerly desire gifts of the Spirit, especially prophecy. For anyone who speaks in a tongue does not speak to people but to God. Indeed, no one understands them; they utter mysteries by the Spirit."

In the Book of Hebrews (11:37–38), the author speaks of biblical personages and prophets who "went about in skins of sheep and goats, destitute, persecuted and mistreated … They wandered in deserts and mountains, living in caves and in holes in the ground." One noteworthy example of such abnormal behavior was Isaiah (20:1–3) who walked about Jerusalem naked for three years in fidelity to the voice of God "as a sign and portent against Egypt and Cush." Another is Jeremiah (Jer. 27:2) who was commanded to fashion a yoke of straps and bars and wear it around his neck. Or, consider Ezekiel, whose odd mannerisms would be worthy of humor, save the dead seriousness of contemporary social, psycho/medical, and legal dynamics. In one passage (Ez. 5:1–4) YHWH tells him to shave his head and beard and then burn a third of the hair inside the city; use a sword to disperse another third about Jerusalem; and scatter the remainder to the wind. What hairs he found clinging to his garment were to be publicly burned as a warning of the fire about to consume Israel. Without pushing the point, were these messengers to perform such "rituals" in the streets of our urban centers, they would normally be corralled by law enforcement, (sometimes) be given a psychiatric examination, perhaps medicated, and, if no space was found in public facilities (or if shelter staff resisted their admittance), arrested and confined.[16]

These brief allusions to Scripture are not intended as proof texts, nor am I a biblical scholar. While these passages suggest that the era in which the texts were written often honored, or at least tolerated, certain behaviors that bordered upon what in the contemporary context would be worthy of clinical, if not penal, intervention, there was an equally prevailing theme that such melodramatic exhibitions were birthed in cosmic malevolence or, perhaps, as a punishment from the Creator. In Deuteronomy (6:5) we hear, "the Lord will smite thee with madness," and the mental collapse of King Saul (1 Sam. 18:10) was thought to have been caused by an evil spirit sent from on high. For their infidelity to the covenant, the prophet Zechariah (12:4) announces to the inhabitants of Jerusalem that divine fury "will strike every horse with panic and its rider with madness." The Pharisees accuse Jesus of casting out devils because they surmised that he gained his power from Satan himself (Mt. 12:24); and there is this most revealing passage in the Gospel of Mark (3:20–21): "Jesus entered a house, and again a crowd gathered, so that he and his disciples were not even able to eat. When his family heard about this, they went to take charge of him, for they said, 'He is out of his mind'."

Obviously, there was at that time no sense of an inner life independent from the gaze and influence of cosmic forces and that is, for our purposes, the essential point. What the Bible gives us, in other words, extrapolated into our own context, is an ambiguous portrait of the psyche whose range and action is dictated not only by external opportunities and legal constraints but also by holy or malignant spiritual powers that were, nonetheless, respected and/or feared as they bordered upon the transcendent and the infinite.

This equivocal approach to the unconventional had equal valence in ancient Greece. Homer's characters, for instance, routinely claim to be compelled, moved, distracted, or deceived by the gods. In fact, the most ancient of the generic terms for the grossly distorted mind in these classic texts is "*entheos*" which translates as "god within."[17] In the "Ion," Socrates comments on Ion's contention that Homer, above all poets, probes most deeply and truthfully into the mysteries of the soul. He writes that lyricists such as Homer are ministers of God, just as the deity "also uses diviners and holy prophets," so that we who hear them may know they speak not from their own store of knowledge but, rather, those "who utter these priceless words in a state of unconsciousness," are but mouthpieces: "God himself is the speaker."[18]

Complementing this, it was widely accepted in both ancient Greek and Roman civilizations that certain persons possessed "exotic powers" and were summoned by the gods to reveal secrets hidden to rational comprehension. They were alternately mediums of "black magic" who could derail the most stable of political and personal itineraries or purveyors of "white magic" with the authority to heal untreatable illness, alter the course of fate, or simply terminate a spell of ill luck.[19]

Among the ancient Egyptians, a medical text from the sixteenth century BCE apprises the attending physician that demonic possession is at the root of madness; a conclusion that an ancient Hindu source, the *Atharva Veda*, duplicates in its advice that sins against the gods suffice to explain the cause of maniacal conduct.[20]

In line with the Homeric affiliation of insanity with surreptitious divinity, Martha Nussbaum writes that in the Greek philosophical tradition certain forms of crazed demeanor are "not only incompatible with [accepted] insight and stability, they are actually necessary for the highest sort of insight and the best kind of stability."[21] For instance, in the "Phaedrus," Plato contends that prophecy, like lunacy, "is the noblest of arts." It is a madness imparted to its ambassadors by Apollo. One designated with this commission has, amidst the "mightiest woes ... come to the rescue of those who are in need." The divine agent is inevitably one who is "truly possessed and duly out of his mind." In fact, Plato states "the sane man is nowhere at all when he enters into rivalry with the madman."[22]

The architects of the Reformation, notably Martin Luther, built their theological and moral edifice on faith, grace, and Scripture—most assuredly not upon reason. The latter was a "whore" when observed in light of spiritual essentials. Since reason was, at best, a "broken reed" in the garden of celestial principles, then the divide between sanity and folly signified little, or at least counted for less than the distinction between those faithful and those rebellious to divine sovereignty.[23] In like manner, Luther's contemporary, Erasmus of Rotterdam, exalted St. Paul's assertion that "God chose the foolish of the world to shame the wise (I Cor. 2:27) and the prayer of Christ who gives thanks "that [God] had conceal'd the Mystery of Salvation from the wise, but revealed it to babes and sucklings, that is to say, Fools" (Mt. 11: 25).[24]

Again, I am not trying to minimize the complexity of the issues that arise with criminal insanity, organic mental handicaps, or the effects of intense trauma and stress that can lead to violent and destructive actions. For instance, there are legitimate cases of those who hear voices or have visual hallucinations who suffer from serious personality disorders but many of those persons are not living in a carceral cage. Nor am I trying to shore up the critique of current criminal justice policy vis-à-vis those considered to be insane by constructing a nostalgic and fanciful Eden of benign tolerance among our pre-modern ancestors. We know that even before the mad were definitively silenced beginning in the eighteenth century, their odd and troublesome mannerisms had bequeathed to them the mantel of the doomed and abandoned lepers.[25] Many of those whose abnormal behavior provoked visceral fear were subject to exorcisms, spurred by the belief in demonic possession, often with catastrophic results.[26] Furthermore, the reader needs no reminder of the fate of many women whose "heretical" opinions and exotic demeanor earned them the terminal and "fiery" accusation of witchcraft, agents of Satanic trickery, and poisoners of pious souls. One need only survey the exotic, if not dreadful, treatments history has left us regarding the subjection of the ill-fated to trepanning (skull boring) and other desperate attempts to free them from their perceived mental maladies to see the truth of the adage that no one (or hardly anyone) stands taller than the generation in which he or she lives.

Despite that necessary reticence, we will see, particularly in the next chapter, that there is a striking difference in worldview between the era we are describing and the one in which we live, although not necessarily in the way the hysterical or confused were treated in discrete historical circumstances. In Catholic nations, for instance, particularly in the Middle Ages, lunatics were shielded under the moral umbrella of the "poor of Christ" and were tended to by healing orders such as the Vincentians and the Brothers and Sisters of Charity. In Spain, Bohemia, and Poland, the latter congregation exercised a comprehensive system of care.[27] Foucault writes that these communities hovered "over madness ... showing it to the world" that we all might learn "a difficult but an essential lesson" about the "guilty innocence" of the irrational in each of us.[28]

By way of summary, Ray Porter gives voice to the ambiguity and necessary paradox that must be honored if we are to construct an historically informed and intellectually and morally inclusive understanding regarding those dwelling outside the domain of common sense:

> Whether or not there ever has been any true dialogue ... between society at large and living mad people ... is a separate and debatable point. But it is certainly true that the utterances of "mad people" were commonly heeded in earlier centuries, not least because the mad were seen as the mouthpieces through whom Otherworldly Powers would speak.[29]

Madness, disease, and confinement

There is some debate, most of it skeptical, about whether the "ship of fools" actually meandered its way along the medieval German countryside, carrying what Foucault terms its "insane cargo" to those settlements where safe harbor was granted. There, the troubled mariners could roam the fields, glean crops, receive the succor of solicitous souls, and even worship at specially consecrated shrines before returning to their "pilgrimage boats" and their "easy wandering existence."[30] Peter Sedgwick categorically denies the existence of such ships while Scull calls Foucault's romantic portrait no more than "a figment of the latter's overly active imagination."[31]

For our purposes, it is not the historical veracity of the specific phenomenon, or Foucault's rendering of it, that compels interest. It is, at the very least, an oblique recognition, born in a long pre-modern history, of a view of authority in which external sanctions and cultural codes were often infused in non-binary fashion with a sense of awe or trepidation before the inexplicable and the miraculous.[32] That is to say that the "insane," despite the misgivings and disquiet they may have provoked, still moved within a "sacred circle."[33] For it was a time, as noted in reference to Catholic charitable institutions, in which divine inscrutability (nominalism in Franciscan theological circles) was regularly invoked to upend the confidently sensible pretensions of the materially and politically dominant. In other words, whether the chronically misunderstood or confused were consigned to floating sanitariums may be up for debate, but there is no doubt that there was, at that time, a general sense in the Middle Ages of divine predilection for the outcast and those being crushed under the wheels of power—for whatever reason.[34]

To extend the maritime metaphor, what commands attention is not whether the ship of fools actually existed; it is that the very "idea" was decommissioned or, rather, refitted. It was overhauled in the moral and epistemological revolution that was forged during the Age of Reason. As for Foucault's bucolic portrait, the archetypal blueprint certainly existed in a shared imagination, or what Jung terms the "collective unconscious"—the real geographical center of the mystic and, often today, the schizophrenic.[35] And it was that capacious archetype, expansive enough to bear the unfathomable and the peculiar, that definitively disappeared below the horizon as a new disciplinary armada was constructed, propelled by fear of the irrational, the metaphysical, and the massive cadre of the hapless and indigent who still moved to the cadence and flow of the now discredited theological opus of a world teeming with enchantment.[36]

A tide was unleashed with the demise of feudalism and the ascendance of mercantilism as a prevailing national policy in sixteenth-century Europe that has yet to recede. Not a tide based on amassing bullion or erasing trade deficits, but upon the mechanisms of the market and, as we will discuss in the next chapter, a new anthropology predicated upon measurable performance and comprehensive systems of evaluation and social control. It was not only the demise of a largely agricultural economy; it was also the wholesale dismissal of the laboring poor, heretofore ensconced within the rigid walls of a feudal structure that kept them at a safe and controlled distance from their overseers. Suddenly, the English highways and towns were flooded with thousands of dismissed feudal retainers and field laborers without domicile or employment. To add to the immediacy of the crisis, the monasteries, traditional sources of sustenance and sanctuary, had been dissolved in the wake of the Protestant Reformation. As one historian notes: "It would be hard to exaggerate the feeling of alarm with which contemporaries, private individuals and public officers, faced this problem."[37]

Typically, English "rogues, vagabonds, idle, loitering, and lewd persons" were subject to sanguinary punishments such as whippings and amputations.[38] While such penalties were never relinquished, in the mid-sixteenth century, at the old Bridewell palace, a workhouse was inaugurated to detain the hordes of the desperate and destitute.[39] Soon, workhouses dotted the entire kingdom. The stated logic was to intervene positively in the lives of vagrants, petty criminals, and the morally corrupt by forcing upon them habits of industry and social propriety.[40] English constables arrested and confined 13,000 of the itinerant needy in 1569 alone.[41] The early bridewells, however, were, by and large, exemplars of neither order nor industriousness; and the logic that governed their operation was driven more by pragmatic fiscal concerns, fear of the uprooted poor, and a utilitarian commitment to deterrence than an impulse to reform "masterless" individuals.[42] While the "able bodied" were provided the tools to learn a trade and pay for their keep, at the same time, in 1572, parliament also sought to further detain a wide array of social misfits with its influential "Acte for the Punishment of Vagabondes, and for Relief of the Poor and Impotent." The bill prescribed the standard penalties for those determined to be culpable in the eyes of the Justices of the Peace. Complementing forced incarceration, an offender was also subject to flogging, ear boring, amputation, and, for repeated failures to conform, execution. Conspicuously absent in the profile of the deviant was the marauding or rapacious predator; that was the purview of the gaol. Rather, the bill aimed to corral a cohort, few of whom were implicated in malicious actions. Instead, emphasis was placed upon "wandering persons using crafty and unlawful games or plays" as well as those "feigning" insights into "Phisonomye, Palmestrye, or other abused Scyences ... and other lyke fantasticall Imaginacions," as well as unlicensed beggars, notably among them starving students from Oxford and Cambridge.[43] We see this confinement of "rabble," to borrow a term from John Irwin, as opposed to serious felons continuing into the eighteenth century.[44] The Vagrancy Act of 1744 accumulated a similarly broad species of offenses as its sixteenth-century counterpart, giving magistrates not only the power to lash beggars, wandering peddlers, gypsies, and others out of step with eighteenth-century social and acquisitive sensibilities, it also stressed confinement for "wandering lunatics" and "all persons wand'ring abroad and lodging in alehouses, barns and houses or in the open air, not giving a good account of themselves."[45] Thus the adverse reaction to the poor was driven not only by their irrelevance to burgeoning capitalist economies but also their susceptibility to visons, spirits, magic, and "elemental forces."[46]

Historical hindsight and its temptation to intellectual pretension is, of course, a caveat not to be taken lightly; a dramatically new summation of the person untethered from obeisance to age-old theological preoccupations and fired into a new materialist universe is quite another. And in this latter perspective, the idea and justification of the workhouse was quickly embraced not only throughout England but also with equal devotion in other locales on the continent such as Holland and the Hanseatic cities of Germany, all awakening to the new economic realities.[47] A large element in its widespread appeal was provided by "bourgeois dissatisfaction with the traditional, noninstitutional response to the indigent."[48] Those who could not contribute in a pragmatic and monetary sense were to be excised from public interchange. In the words of the eminent jurist, William Blackstone, the poor had to be arrested, prosecuted, and confined for the theft of rabbits, not only because it was injurious to the sporting interests of the gentry, but also to prevent "low and indigent persons" from failing to busy themselves with "proper employments and callings."[49]

In his study of prison writing in the wake of the English Reformation, Thomas Freeman speaks of the decisive shift in the attitudes toward the poor that we have been describing. In consequence, the sturdy seeds of a perception were planted in the sixteenth century, flourished in the mid-eighteenth century, and still bear fruit today: "that crime is largely caused by the poor." The result, as we have seen, was that since the impoverished were portrayed as a social threat "*tout court*," "then it was a social necessity to provide places where the poor (particularly vagrants, but also those who were rebellious or refractory) could be educated out of their wicked ways and trained to be productive members of society."[50]

Zygmunt Bauman sees in the repressive measures we have been discussing the birth of the "absolutist state" with its imposed universality; one driven by a "crusade against vulgar, beastly, superstitious habits" in obeisance to a cultural ideology wherein hegemonic dominance was portrayed in the guise of "the superior way of life" whose carriers were "to be emulated by all."[51]

What is decidedly significant in the pivotal historical approach to the marginal that we are describing is that incarceration, for the first time in a systematic sense, found its impetus not from a focus upon direct material and bodily harm but upon the distinction between the productive and the non-productive.[52] In Foucault's rendering, the workhouse brought into a complex unity this distinctly adverse reaction to poverty and aid to the penniless and idiosyncratic. It instituted "new forms of reaction to the economic problems of unemployment and idleness, a new ethic of work."[53] Furthermore, the new disciplinary approach, so imbued with dread not only of the lower classes but also of their "fantasticall imaginacions," fell under the rigid "exactitude of a social order, imposed from without and ... by force."[54] It was, in its own way, an optimistic judicial logic, emboldened by the claim that such aggressive tactics, in spite of the masses unprepared or otherwise unsuited for "proper employments," would "gradually restore the minds of maniacs to the light of truth."[55]

And this measurement of human worth and of human development, predicated upon productive capacity and the institutionalization of the socially and economically problematic, is the crux of what I want to work with throughout this volume. It was in that newly fashioned milieu that the image of the tranquil or even troubled "madman" living in a world of supernatural voices and visions was definitively transformed, not on a person-to-person basis, or even in a specific institutional regimen, but in a system-wide designation of deviance. The shadow of lunacy cast by the ranks of the insignificant and the intimidating fell upon a public (just as it does today) aggressively determined to banish its presence. The plight of the former had devolved from "a vague, culturally defined phenomenon … into a condition that could be authoritatively diagnosed, certified, and dealt with by a group of legally recognized experts."[56]

John Lofland has examined in detail the etiology of the concept of deviance; and while the term in its present sociological attire was absent in the period of which we speak, the hallmarks of the notion were startlingly evident: a moniker of cognitive incapacity and "inappropriate behavior" attributed to individuals and "loosely organized groups" with little social clout, magnified by a pronounced fear among a "well organized, sizable minority or majority who have a large amount of power."[57]

Despite John Witte's claim that the uncoupling of law and punishment from all ties to religious principles removed any transcendent foundation for criminal law and replaced it with utilitarian and self-defensive visions that deny most people's sense of why law is written and obeyed in the first place, the ancient rite of excommunication was decisively reconfigured, not in terms of orthodox belief and ritual practice, but in fealty to the new liturgy of production, commerce, and the dismissal of the unproductive.[58] It was into these spaces "that madness would appear and soon expand until it had annexed them."[59]

The growth of and crisis within psychiatric care

The rise and fall of moral treatment

The foregoing has left us with an aberrant portrait of those unconventional souls lumped together in a spectacle of stigma and dismay. What became and remains of central significance is the role of physicians in verifying socioeconomic fears and the resultant movement to forcibly quarantine the "insane" by turning those fears into medical facts. Foucault claims that what was decisive in the transition of madness from a metaphysical quandary into an exhibition of chronic a-sociability was the role of "*homo medicus*" who "was not called into the world of confinement as an *arbiter*, to divide what was crime from what was madness, what was evil from what was illness, but rather as a *guardian*, to protect others from the vague danger that exuded through the walls of confinement."[60]

Let me begin with those who tried to circumvent the popular and professional opinion that those caught in the nets of a suspicious, or better, threatened culture of "sanity" and financial self-interest were to be summarily demoted and dismissed. The former still believed that the "insane" were capable of full integration into the world of acceptable social etiquette *sans* the punitive mandate. Their efforts were predicated upon a claim that will occupy us consistently in our study, namely, their determination, to varying degrees, to see the politics of sanity as a moral, or what can be termed a metaethical, issue. For within their, ultimately failed, plea for tolerance for the "other" was the belief that the rejected were, in the first place, human beings with the innate capacity to respond warmly and positively to care and compassionate presence. Perhaps Jaspers captures best the approach of the individuals we will briefly survey: "[T]he more we reduce [those labeled as mentally ill] to what is typical and normative the more we realize there is something hidden in every human individual which defies recognition. We have to be content with partial knowledge of an infinity which we cannot exhaust."[61]

Phillipe Pinel assumed control of the French asylums of Bicetre and Salpetriere in 1793. He wrote passionately of the effects of the institutional confinement he had witnessed upon those whose diagnostic forecast was not a prescription for recovery but, far too often, a sentence of death: "The managers of those [public] institutions, who are frequently men of little knowledge and less humanity, have been permitted to exercise towards their innocent prisoners a most arbitrary system of cruelty and violence."[62]

His medical knowledge, his experience, not to mention his conscience, prompted him to alter the treatment patients would receive under his supervision. While a strict disciplinarian in the spirit of the materialism of the times and its belief in re-socialization, he observed that the anger and surliness of many of those he treated upon their arrival (thinking here of the involuntary prophet) was the result not of organic malfunction but callous abuse.[63]

At the same time, he catalogued the repeated benefits of kindness and patience, finding that the cure of many deemed invincibly unstable was directly related to the degree of dignity and ontological worth extended to them. He wrote that those transferred to his institution

and represented upon their arrival as more than commonly furious and dangerous, rendered so no doubt by severe treatment, have, upon being received with affability, soothed by consolation and sympathy, and encouraged to expect a happier lot, suddenly subsided into a placid calmness, to which has succeeded a rapid convalescence.[64]

Put simply, he found that the exclusive deployment of a moral regimen "gives weight to the supposition, that, in a majority of instances, there is no organic lesion of the brain nor of the cranium."[65]

Meanwhile, in England, William Tuke, a devout Quaker who had observed first-hand the deeply flawed and disturbing protocols forced upon members of his congregation who had been forcibly institutionalized, opened the York Retreat in 1796 with a moral perspective and set of beliefs parallel to those of Pinel. His grandson, Samuel, assumed directorship of the Retreat shortly thereafter and continued to engage in his grandfather's mission. The younger Tuke wrote that the knowledge he gained from working with the patients diverted from the public facilities "demonstrated, beyond all contradiction, the superior efficacy, both in respect of cure and security, of a mild system of treatment in all cases of mental disorder."[66] He further asserted that perhaps the strongest evidence of the rectitude of "benevolent affections" was the degree of warmth evinced from the patients when approached with the care each human being deserves.[67]

His theological commitments were very much a part of his motivation and methodology; a point worth emphasizing as it hearkens to a time when those functioning outside the realm of common sense were seen to be in the grip of forces to be honored, if not necessarily understood, and touched by what Jaspers points to as a "hidden ... infinity which we cannot exhaust." Tuke writes that those of his contemporaries pursuing a more punitive approach would "do well to reflect on the awful responsibility which attaches to their conduct." He then adds: "Let us all constantly remember, that there is a Being, to whose eye darkness is light; who sees the inmost recesses of the dungeon, and who has declared: 'For the sighing of the poor, and the crying of the needy, I will arise.'"[68]

The efforts of Pinel and Tuke were not ignored on the other side of the Atlantic. The "corporate" institutions constructed in the United States in the early nineteenth century reflected their inspiration. For example, the Friends' Asylum in Pennsylvania was patterned upon the York Retreat after its founder, Thomas Scattergood, had visited that facility.[69] Also, in the person of Dorothea Dix, mentally ill men and women confined in "cages, closets, stalls, pens! Chained, naked, beaten with rods [and] lashed into obedience" found a tireless champion.[70]

Another of the asylums, the Hartford Retreat (1824), also affirmed the benefits of kindly treatment toward its residents. However, its first superintendent, Eli Todd, also balanced the curative regimen with an equal emphasis on medical intervention, a practice that was emulated by the managers of other establishments. According to Heather Vacek, physicians believed that addressing presumed somatic imbalances cultivated the ground upon which moral influences could have their most desired effect.[71] Of note, clergy were apt to take the same view of frontloading physical remedies over moral or spiritual ones. The sermon of a local minister at the dedication of the Hartford Retreat lauded the replacement of the religious miracle with the skill of the physician. He stated the while "the insane found a safe retreat in Christ" the "power to cure insanity through miraculous means [was] now withdrawn" with only natural means needed to perform the same task.[72]

This bicameral approach planted a worm in the apple of a unified moral methodology, one that steadily began to eat away at its appeal. Of interest for the current treatment regimen, the resumption of an assertive corporal intervention and the prophylactics that began to be employed by sanitorium staff were more and more accompanied by the employment of a range of aggressive medications, particularly "the growing reliance on opium and morphine that became characteristic of American asylum practice."[73]

David Rothman's study of the nascence of curative detention centers in the Jacksonian era bears witness to the cultural dynamic that fused with the medicalization and, in many aspects, criminalization of insanity, and soon overwhelmed the desires of the few who refused to succumb to what soon became a visceral public sense of alarm with an accompanying cry for increased confinement. He writes, reminiscent of the panic that seized the English upper class at the sight of throngs of displaced feudal laborers, that "discussions of insanity, like those of crime, conveyed a heightened, almost hysterical sense of peril, with the very safety of the republic and its citizens at stake."[74]

The same fate of which Rothman speaks befell the efforts of erstwhile reformers in Europe, although in a few visionary superintendents, such as William Connolly, the sensitivity and loatheness to reduce the identification of the hospitalized with mental infirmity continued into the 1850s.[75] It is not possible to verify the claims of Pinel, Tuke, and later Connolly, that tolerant and compassionate accompaniment revealed that most of their patients suffered from the effects of maltreatment rather than organic handicaps. What we do know is that the managers of other public institutions (wedded to a primarily biological regimen) were dismayed at what they perceived as the unconvincing lack of similar positive outcomes (there is an irony there that I will leave the reader to possibly entertain).

The nail that effectively sealed the coffin of the moral strategy was driven in the US in 1844, when the superintendents of 13 asylums formed the Association of Medical Superintendents of American Institutions for the Insane (AMSAII). We noted that attempts to balance care and curative intervention—the announced method of the new association—inevitably eroded the former and elevated the latter with a regimen heavily dependent upon the use of sedatives and narcotics. Robert Whitaker writes that asylum physicians used "mild cathartics, bloodletting on occasion, and various drugs—most notably morphine and opium—to sedate patients. Their use of such chemical 'restraints,' in turn, made them more receptive to the use of physical restraints, which they increasingly turned to as their asylums became more crowded."[76]

As a result, the corporate facilities, constructed with such reformist zeal, gradually returned, as Joel and Ian Gold point out, to their former function as "warehouses for the chronically ill ... whose task was not to cure but to keep the sick and the sedated, out of sight, and (because madness was now thought to be hereditary) celibate." They conclude: "Conditions in many of the asylums were again simply dreadful."[77] From Scull's viewpoint, studies of such institutions "all revealed a depressingly similar feature." Far from the quest to restore their inhabitants to social acceptability, they descended into simply a "disabling, custodial function."[78] While Vacek notes that both public and professional perceptions of madness came to surround "the afflicted with disgrace." And with the new emphases on hereditary and other destabilizing somatic factors now fully in play, and with definitive cures still lodged in a seemingly ill-founded optimism, she writes that "the chronically ill seemed doomed."[79]

Thus, moral treatment morphed into the default response that marked its immediate predecessors, and, by and large, its successors down to this day: another species of mandatory detention, a cloak over a subliminally frightening specter, "a more thorough-going form of repression."[80] Rothman sums up the seismic shift, strengthened now with the explicit sanction of remedial "experts," that lends credence to the overall thrust of our study. He concludes that "the asylum system was highly regimented and repressive ... [overseen by medical superintendents] carrying out the logic of a theory of deviancy ... in a tightly organized and rigid environment ... Their program did resemble that of the penitentiary."[81]

Mental illness as pathology

Once medical diagnoses both modeled and became a model for an anxious and wary public, a strictly materialist, and increasingly biological, response was all that remained to cope with the mentally and emotionally peculiar. The work of the Scottish physician, William Cullen, was highly instrumental in this regard. He insisted that cognitive disorders were diseases of the nervous system. It was he who deployed the term "neurosis" to designate such states. He forwarded the theory "that the 'nerve fluid' by which the brain functioned might be electrical and that mental disorders might come about by nervous over—or under—excitation."[82] Showing the influence of his empiricist predecessor, John Locke, he claimed that the effect of these neuroses was a psychological one, " 'a hurried association of ideas' producing 'false judgement'—and under the influence of Cullen's views, the *mind* of the mental patient came to the fore in medical thinking about insanity and its treatment."[83]

While this doctrinal shift mitigated the strictly punitive response that had, in Porter's words, "likened the mad to brutes," it categorized those labeled as insane as infants, incapable on their own of rational and ethical deduction. Thus, like the education of children, they should be housed in facilities—recall the stated function of the workhouse—that they might be "reconditioned for civilized life."[84] Such "total institutions," predicated upon the behaviorist assumption that external sensations were, using Locke's words, the substance of the preternaturally "empty cabinet" of the psyche, could exact a nearly complete measure of control over the social life of the patient by overseeing the full range of sensual stimuli.[85]

A noteworthy example of this emphasis on a Lockean protocol of mental rehabilitation through aggressive intervention is seen in Benjamin Rush, a signer of the US Declaration of Independence and Surgeon General of the Army during the War of Independence. Rush studied medicine in Edinburgh and came under the influence of William Cullen. Like his mentor, Rush understood mental impairment as the fruit of impediments in the nervous or vascular system. Working at the Philadelphia Hospital for the Insane, he devised a series of experiments to counter the effects of assumed neural handicaps. He frequently practiced blood-letting, the ingestion of mercury to purge the body, the tranquilizing chair whose aim was to pacify patients in the throes of hysteria (they were affixed to the chair with their heads immobilized until they had been calmed and their mania had subsided), and engineered a "gyrator" that would whirl the distressed subject at a high speed, forcing blood into the brain and inducing what was assumed to be a normal or acceptable state of cognition. Vacek affirms the profound influence of Enlightenment empiricism on his thought and under his tutelage madness in America was further transformed from a religious or moral phenomenon to a "treatable" medical one.[86]

Such a coercive methodology had a *prima facie* appeal as long as lunacy could be recognized as such, rather than simply a moniker for the homeless wanderer or outlandish character in an economy of manufacture and gain. However, again referencing Porter, if publicly transparent mannerisms such as looking, acting, and talking "crazy" were synonymous with persistent abnormality, the sanction to remove such to be "reconditioned," or at least kept at an enclosed distance, would be easily affirmed, or perhaps even be accomplished, by any competent and dedicated observer (say, a family member). However, one of the tenets of psychiatry, the domain of the "alienist," as practitioners were then called, was the conviction that insanity "could be fearsomely latent, biding its time," only capable of being detected by the trained medical professional.[87] Thus, institutionalization and forceful intrusion into the day to day functioning of the suspected lunatic was, in one way or the other, the reaction most frequently engaged.

I will not weary the reader with a detailed psychiatric history, readily available in multiple studies, a number of which were consulted for this book, but the waning of a humanist-cum-therapeutic treatment regimen with the spread of public institutions continued to be progressively undermined as a bevy of further scientific theories began to delve more authoritatively and convincingly into deviations in brain function as the determining cause of mental illness as opposed to social, moral, or, for that matter, spiritual conditions.

Having said that, a few historical notes are necessary. In the late eighteenth century, Emil Kraepelin, a German psychiatrist, deemed "contemporary psychiatry's patron saint" who "laid the foundations upon which … biological psychiatry was later built," made significant strides in the categorization of the state of mental delirium.[88] He maintained that the latter consisted of "dementia praecox," an early onset (praecox) and progressive cognitive deterioration (dementia). Noteworthy for our study as it unfolds is the identification of this condition with hallucinations, delusions, and general emotional inadaptability.[89]

The origin of the term "schizophrenia" was left to Kraepelin's successor, Eugen Bleuler, who like the former, had noted the variety of maladies, especially rational disorientation, displayed by patients so diagnosed. However, Bleuler took Kraepelin one step further in trying to specify a common denominator or essential property that would tie the types together. He found this metaphorical concept in what he called the "breaking of associative threads."[90] Of interest for our purposes is that summation varies little from the social experience of both the voluntary prophet—the adamant and reviled public critic of the status quo—and the involuntary prophet, often the schizophrenic, perpetually out of stride in the march of normalcy.

The impact of the work of Kraepelin and Bleuler has been profound on the psychiatric community up to our own day, regarding both early inception and the symptoms of dementia such as attunement to voices, susceptibility to imaginative visions, and other stimuli not reducible to empirical detection or measurement. It has also helped solidify a general aura of actual or latent criminality that has surrounded and continues to surround those determined to be intellectually handicapped.

Regarding initial onset and the correlation of psychosis with childhood socialization forwarded by both Kraepelin and Bleuler, one contemporary study notes the influence of Michael Gottfredson and Travis Hirschi's influential monograph that emphasizes the lack of self-control in the formative years as the most consistent factor in predicting future criminal misbehavior. What is noteworthy here is the theory of psychic abnormality occurring early in the life course and, more relevant for our study, affixing it to an aberrant model of human development: "Many psychiatric disorders emerge early in life ... For example, most impulse control disorders ... begin in childhood ... [T]he idea is consistent with Gottfredson and Hirschi's general theory of crime."[91]

An influential essay by Terrie Moffit continues the association of antisocial behavior in toddlerhood not only with life-course persistent illegal activity but also with "subtle dysfunctions of the nervous system." He cites a study positing that a conviction for acts of violence in their early 20s "is characteristic of almost all men who become diagnosed with antisocial (psychopathic) personality disorder."[92] He adds that the prognosis for such persons "is bleak," specifically due to the evidence of longitudinal studies that assert the presence of verbal and executive neuropsychological deficits associated with aberrant behavior. Verbal deficits "of antisocial children are pervasive, affecting receptive listening and reading, problem solving, expressive speech and writing, and memory." Executive deficits are identified in conjunction with cognitive ability and are related to "inattention and impulsivity."[93]

It is worthwhile at this juncture to call to mind an insightful study by Ian Loader in which he turns the tables on "self-control" theory and its relation to early childhood disfunction. He insists that a common and disturbing example of the lack of self-control, or the presence of "impulse control disorder," is evidenced in the draconian policy of summarily judging, silencing, and carting away to prison overwhelming numbers of men and women considered threatening to the chimerical public and political desire for instant solutions to unreal expectations for blanket protection and security.[94] The agents and supporters of vehement repressive measures are certain that the reckless actions that turn the child into a lawbreaker and the lawbreaker into an inmate are logically explicable and the ensuing punishments justifiable. Never put to question is their own reckless punitive impulsiveness that has turned America and, to a lesser but significant extent, Great Britain into world leaders in imprisonment, and imprisonment more and more into a euphemism for the punishment of the insane.[95]

Jock Young surveys the "slash and burn" politics of sanity in parallel terms. It assumes, erroneously, that offenders are like buckets that have "sprung a leak," and that the social structure itself is guiltless in its impact upon those without leverage who rail against the harsh constraints imposed against their flourishing.[96] Moreover, he upbraids the "English upper classes" for their pretense of loyalty to what conservatives in America call "family values." He caustically points to the "institutionalized practice of 'broken' homes" in which children are typically ushered by their parents to prep and finishing schools; a custom repeatedly found in the "Royal Family with its growing tendency to live in separate palaces." Both, he argues, are just as likely as poor families "to produce a prodigious crop of delinquents."[97]

Concerning Kraepelin and Bleuler's second signal of psychosis, dementia, and its penchant for believing in acoustic and visual revelations, one contemporary psychiatrist terms those in its grip to be guilty of "thought insertion." He describes the condition as a misleading "delusion" that is typically associated with "disorders such as alien voices, thought-withdrawal, and so-called passivity experiences." However, once the "victim" (or, perhaps, prophet) posits the encounter, that person "is absolutely convinced" and "cannot be dissuaded" from its unorthodox conclusion.[98] Another study attests: "Psychosis is described as a disorganization of thoughts and emotional responses to reality. Common symptoms include significant changes in behaviour, social isolation, feelings of suspicion, unusual beliefs, hearing voices, seeing things ... The process of becoming psychotic creates profound psychological changes that are frightening."[99] For Eric Kandel, schizophrenia proceeds from a strictly neural disorder that features chaotic thought sequences that detach "a person from reality, leading to altered perceptions and behavior, such as hallucinations and delusions." Such hallucinations "can be visual or auditory. Auditory hallucinations are very troubling: patients hear voices."[100]

Combining the two perspectives (early onset and dementia), we see the downward spiral in which an effect is looking for a recognizable, scientifically verifiable cause. In a disenchanted world, medical experts confronting the bizarre and uncomfortable (almost without fail attached to the social standing of the problematic person), reinforce the common determination, perhaps even at this point a social construction, that such "delusions" exist as actual or latent criminal indicators requiring the intervention of the psychiatrist and, all too commonly, the judge and the jailer. Bauman brings these ideas into systemic focus in his observation that in the modern bureaucratic state, the intellectual has been supplanted by the expert. And foremost among the "expert-intensive techniques" are those obsessed with "panoptic social control," among which he includes surveillance, correction, medicalization, psychiatrization, and servicing the legal/penal system.[101]

I will close this section on welding "out of body" experiences and the mental states they engender with a disreputable, deleterious, and deviant diagnosis with these thoughts from Anne Harrington. She contends that the attempt of late nineteenth-century researchers such as Kraepelin to locate questionable cerebral function solely within the biological realm was erroneous because he and his successors "were not only early versions of ourselves, but also because it failed." Even Kraepelin himself eventually came to recognize this. However, by that time, the biological wheel had been set in motion. Still, she adds that "those who pursued this project 'bet' on anatomy and lost" and their failure "cast a long shadow" over psychiatric practice. She further notes, as we will discuss shortly, that "some clinicians, including a number of neurologists, responded by turning to nonbiological understandings of mental disorders, including psychoanalytic ones." These, however, have been largely superseded by the exclusively organic wing of psychiatry which "was left in a state of disarray and increasingly pursued a hodgepodge of theories and projects, many of which, in hindsight, look both ill-considered and incautious."[102]

Biology, psychotherapy, and the fate of the mentally handicapped

My intent in the following brief survey of psychoanalytic responses to various paranormal events is not necessarily to pit one remedial strategy against another, since both medical and therapeutic responses are still very much in play in the treatment of cognitive or emotional unrest. There are, however, several caveats that are germane to what I am trying to do in this volume that will condition my report. The first of which is that the psychic maladies of the poor, in the great majority of instances, disqualify them economically from psychological analysis since, in deference to the ongoing prevalence of strictly medical protocols, the robust resources of the former tradition have largely been funneled into private consultations with paying customers.[103] The patients that licensed counselors have taken under their wing are, by and large, not categorized with the stigmatic and, often, class-influenced branding of psychosis or schizophrenia that readily mechanizes the forces of social control to direct its bearer—thinly cloaked to hide the deviant label—to the nearest police lockup. Rather, as pointed out in the Introduction, the personal anxieties and neuroses of the well-to-do are normally addressed in comfortable professional suites, various genres of support groups, or in the domestic setting.

A second caveat is that this privatization of care, as noted earlier, has been exaggerated by the wholesale shuttering of public institutions whose announced aim was, for better or worse, a more integrated approach to remedy objectionable mental states. As has been pointed out, a jail sentence is more and more the assumed response to the impoverished, many of them wandering and begging in the streets, who have been lumped into the troubled category. However, as a further consequence, there is a paucity of neurological support services in the vast gulag of America's jail and prison empire.[104] The National Alliance of Mental Illness (NAMI) estimates that 83 percent of prisoners so classified lack access to the treatments they need. Those treatments in turn are "at best, a bottle of pills and a referral when they are released, leading to a revolving door of arrests and short-term incarceration with no real improvement in the person's underlying mental health."[105] Alisa Roth reports that most American prisons are in rural areas with an inadequate number of competent professionals. Quoting one doctor: "No one who went to medical school said, 'I want to incur this much debt and spend my life working in prisons.'"[106] She then adds that an alarming number of those who staff penal institutions have been previously reprimanded for delinquent treatment procedures; prison being the only available venue wherein they can engage in clinical practice.[107] The situation in Great Britain is equally disturbing. Health-care standards established by the National Health Service require that services for detainees diagnosed with mental distress be performed by a "doctor who is psychiatrically qualified," meaning that the physician's name must appear on the relevant specialist register. Available data suggest that this is far from the case. In a survey of 13 prisons, the authors of one study relate that not one of the doctors practicing there met this standard.[108]

Where such services are provided, they are often tainted either by the stultifying effects of psychotropic drugs, or by the frequent servitude of prison psychologists to a host of rehabilitative initiatives that reinforce the malformed label of the incarcerated and shape their interventions not to the good of the specific client but to his or her acquiescence to the dominant economic and social hierarchy. We will investigate this in greater detail in Chapter 3; but, briefly stated, psychological interventions are regularly judged to be successful if the patient steers clear of what are commonly called criminogenic tendencies (for example, lack of self-control). For those who fail to embrace, or at least project, both an understanding of and a behavioral assent to the standards established by program administrators to evaluate compliance and "rehabilitation," the asocial label is reinforced, and the participant is carted back to his or her cell.

Third, even acknowledging the vast resources that the psychological tradition has accumulated over the decades, psychoanalysis, in many of its approaches to mental duress, is often incapable of attending to the sort of transcendent or mystical experiences that convert ordinary persons into prophetic mouthpieces. One study contends that "there is an inclination among psychoanalysts to conclude that various psychopathological conditions are related to religious involvement."[109] For John Swinton, therapists and psychiatrists tend to "regard spirituality and religion as, at best, cultural noise to be respected but not addressed directly, or at worst pathological thinking that requires modification."[110] Extending this bias to social scientists generally, Rodney Stark notes that when he and his coauthor, William Bainbridge, compiled research on mystical experience, they found in conversation with numerous colleagues in the human sciences that "the psychopathological interpretation was the overwhelming favorite, with conscious fraud treated as the only possible alternative."[111]

Philip Rieff's commentary upon this ingrained bias is worth noting. He sees the preeminent task of most analysts as an attempt to provide the tools to contravene the exaggerated sense of loneliness and alienation experienced by so many rather than to emphasize "an effective sense of communion" made possible by "rendering the inner life serviceable to the outer." In line with the animus demonstrated in the citations just provided, he sees the discipline more and more geared "to protect the outer life against further encroachments from the inner."[112]

Fourth, neither does therapeutic training tend to urge its clinicians to pay heed to the societal factors that so often induce psychic conditions that provoke a spontaneous rejection of the prevailing political and economic consensus that I maintain is the function and burden of the prophet.

These limitations are not meant to diminish the importance of the classic texts in psychoanalysis, particularly those of Freud and Jung. In spite of works written by the former that sought to reduce religious belief and, by extension, direct mystical experience (remembering Stark and Bainbridge) to inherent pathology, conscious fraud or, in his terminology, neurotic attachment to the "father" figure, he always maintained "a sober vision" of the human being caught at the edge of the competing forces of the external culture and internal instincts and that the fully mature person had "the trained capacity to keep the negotiations from breaking down."[113] An example of this perspective, and parenthetically, its disharmony from strict somatic renderings of human motivation and action, is seen in Freud's contention of the "essential" nature of instinctual drives. These "unconscious mental processes are in themselves 'timeless.' That is to say, to begin with: they are not arranged chronologically, time alters nothing in them, nor can the idea of time be applied to them."[114] And, in his view, the excessively materialist rendering of conduct that is "out of the ordinary" reveals as much about the projection of the analyst as it does about the misshapen perception of the patient. For those who "bet on biology," to use Harrington's words, Freud astutely suggests that there

> will be a tendency to treat [those under analysis] as though they were acting not from within but from without, in order for it to be possible to apply against them the defensive measures of the barrier against stimuli. This is the origin of projection, for which so important a part is reserved in the production of pathological states.[115]

This is not to suggest that Freud was dismissive of the contributions of natural science to help perceive the nature and even treatment of patterns of action induced by experiences of trauma or hysteria: "Biology is truly a realm of limitless possibilities; we have the most surprising revelations to expect from it, and cannot conjecture what answers it will offer in some decades to the questions we have put to it."[116] Rather, he regularly utilized the term "metapsychology" to synthesize the complex union of factors, each with its own integrity, that both those under scrutiny and the clinician must honor to approximate psychic wholeness, with the inner, instinctual forces assuming the most determinative, but by no means only, role:[117] "Naturally the excitations coming from within will, in conformity with their intensity and other qualitative characteristics ... be more proportionate to the mode of operation of the system than the stimuli streaming in from the outer world."[118]

The foregoing is only a drop in the river of Freud's vast and influential corpus, but, from my perspective, it is to be honored. This is especially due to its explicit recognition that "timeless" drives that can neither be expunged, nor reduced to epiphenomena, nor "welded into the comprehensive unity of the ego," are the real aim of the therapist whose task is to enable a patient to uncover, own, and integrate unconscious impulses that must neither be denied nor repressed lest they be reproduced continually and, in one way or another, destructively.[119]

Jung complements and exceeds Freud's focus on the inner life as integral and determinative of one's appropriation of and response to outer stimuli. As most know, the two, once close colleagues, parted ways not over the supervening role of the unconscious, but over the content of the instinctual drives, with Freud relying almost exclusively on the Oedipal myth and that of the murder of the primal father. Jung, on the other hand, developed an extensive catalogue of archetypal symbols and susceptibilities that do not owe their existence "to personal experience and consequently [are] not a personal acquisition." They are "definite forms in the psyche which seem to be present always and everywhere."[120] For him, these primal symbols represent the basic truths of the universe.

Such spiritual forces, in his estimation, inhabit the deepest part of the psyche and control us far more than we control them. They have the capacity to "seize" and "possess" an aspirant or, merely, as Jung points out, a simple "carpet weaver," referring to St. Paul, with neither knowledge of nor intent to communicate with them.[121] And it is these inner instincts and transcendent realities that provide the very substance of the mysterious insights that people who encounter such powers possess.

Jung, himself, is a most relevant case in point of one who was on numerous occasions overtaken by sudden revelations of a deeply spiritual nature. The effects upon him were dramatic, certainly providing fodder for the flames of discontent that consumed his relationship with Freud. He compares "the spirit of this time" that only concerns itself with "use and value" with another spirit "which rules the depths of everything contemporary." And while he admits that he was once in the throes of that pragmatic spirit, that other spirit "from time immemorial" "forces me nevertheless to speak, beyond justification, use, and meaning."[122]

In Jung's system, the unconscious has preserved these "primitive characteristics" that so affected him and that form "part of the original mind." These archetypal myths and symbols often appear in the frequently peculiar content of dreams "as if the unconscious sought to bring back all the old things from which the mind freed itself as it evolved." However, without acknowledgment of their reality and power, they summon "resistance, even fear." This reflexive dismissal of the commonly terrifying revelations produced by unmediated symbols must be faced resolutely for "the more they are repressed, the more they spread through the whole personality in the form of neurosis."[123]

Despite the warnings that Jung presents, we have seen that active acknowledgment and expression of the messages such primal and perennial forces convey to certain types of individuals, many of whom I am depicting as voluntary or involuntary prophets, are viewed as explicit signs of cognitive and emotional failure. Such a position, tenaciously held by the medical materialist or strict behaviorist, rapidly summons the attending authoritative judgments that have deposed so many into caverns of isolation with, oftentimes, equally aggressive strategies to restore them to their "right minds."

Jung readily acknowledges that for those allied to a rigorous scientific mindset, such phenomena "are a nuisance because they cannot be formulated in a way that is satisfactory to the intellect and logic." In fact, as he states, the "academic psychologist is perfectly free to dismiss [them]." However, he warns that if any psychologist is to treat patients effectively, he or she "comes up against these realities as hard facts."[124]

Alternately, the shedding of ego defenses and attentiveness to the deepest part of the self enables the ego to be illuminated "by knowledge of the existence of psychic dimensions beyond its own reality." These intimations of and encounters with the collective unconscious are, I believe, the wellspring of the prophetic. Such transcendent moments "include intimations of realms of experience that transcend the familiar textures of psychic encounter." Something totally other has come to us, "permitting us to be part of another life," a state of union that Jung calls the "imago."[125] These arcane experiences enable one to uncover the hidden emotional aspect of what is truly occurring and thus help compensate for the egoic attempt to master or expel such intimations and impulses: "This new mixture shifts the center of gravity from ego to Self. A new center grows in consciousness that joins parts that had been split apart."[126]

In this short summary of the two most influential progenitors of the psychotherapeutic discipline, we see that internal, archaic, and persistent forces have a decided impact on a person's ability to navigate the life course free of fear, projection, and neurosis. It is the human task to live at the meeting point of the inner and outer worlds, understanding the hidden and immense power of internal instincts or archetypes in shaping the psyche and its relation to the experiential milieu. This is by no means a suggestion that contemporary practitioners of the discipline rely on these classical approaches. In fact, according to Rieff, remembering the implicit bias of many trained in the sciences against any recognition, let alone honoring, of the metaphysical, "current systems of therapeutic control" function in seeking to limit "the area of spontaneity" and are decidedly "anti-instinctual." They are called "therapeutic" "because the controls are intended to preserve a certain established level of adequacy in the social functioning of the individual."[127]

In either case, as observed in the qualifications at the beginning of this section, the resources appreciative of an a-priori, universal psychic foundation—what in spiritual terminology might be termed the "numinous"—have either been directed to the psychological well-being of affluent clients, ignored by new generations of therapists, or, as we have already made known, fallen afoul of the current biological paradigm. As Jacques Lacan articulates, there is now little resistance to imperial medical dogma. Where there were once limits to its activity, these limits "no longer depend upon anything more than the numerical strength by which its presence is measured on the social scale."[128]

A case of the dismissal, indeed inherent dangers, of turning to therapeutic intervention in a universe dominated by strictly pragmatic categories is revealed in the story of Daniel Senior. He was aware of unhealthy, unconscious sexual drives and desired to enter therapy even before being incarcerated. However, he writes: "I was worried that prosecution would find out … and they would deem me crazy and that would negatively affect my sentencing."[129] One study helps substantiate the claimant's story of the power of medical testimony to diminish the validity of other remedial sources: "Mental health experts who testify at trial use relevant disorders listed in the DSM [Diagnostic and Statistical Manual] and the defendant's symptoms as [definitive] evidence about the defendant's mental state."[130]

Biology, drugs, and deviance

Whatever relevance the foregoing approaches may have had or continue to have for specific practitioners and clients, a growing number of therapists and psychiatrists came to concur that Freudian and, to a lesser extent, Jungian leadership "had presided over a slow train wreck."[131] By the 1970s, those voices of dissent, strengthened by the continued push provided by the ideas of Kraepelin and other innovators in biological psychiatry, fully overhauled treatment initiatives into those dominated by medical fact and physical remedies to the point that it began to appear certain that "there can be no twisted thought without a twisted molecule."[132]

Of course, as we have already seen, aggressive incursion upon and into the bodies of suspected "lunatics" was hardly a new idea. However, as Scull points out, despite the sometimes crude curative methods of the past such as trepanning or Rush's gyrator and tranquilizing chair, it was the twentieth century that displayed the "most startling examples of the psychiatric profession's predilection for physical treatments," ranging from mosquito therapy through Metrazol-induced seizures, insulin comas, electroshock treatment, lobotomies, and other attempts to blame the brain for the outbreak of unconventional and troubling behavior.[133]

None of these "cures," however, was more widespread or aggressive in both its distribution and effects than the return to one of the earliest strategies to pacify unruly or bewildered patients: drugs. We have already noted the common use of opium and morphine in the early American asylums. While the mollifying effects of those medications, and later those of barbiturates, were unquestioned in their function as "managerial tools," American psychiatry found no scientific justification for their use as antidotes for suspected cerebral malfunction.[134]

All of that changed in the 1950s with the unveiling of Chlorpromazine (Thorazine). Pharmaceutical companies rapidly foresaw the immense market value of a medication that seemed not only to counteract the effects of major psychological maladies such as schizophrenia, depression, and mood disorders but also, due to its impact on neural transmitters, reconfigure the brain in a way that promised to aid in overcoming the adverse effects of those conditions.[135] After only one year of approval by the Food and Drug Administration, the company that was awarded the patent, Smith, Kline, & French, saw its sales rise by one third. After ten years, approximately 50 million prescriptions had been filled and the corporation's profit margins doubled three times in a period of 15 years.[136] It may thus come as no surprise to the reader that more money is spent developing, testing, and analyzing psychopharmacological drugs than in any other area of psychiatry.[137]

Advertising campaigns developed to promote Thorazine and other medications, aware of the immense revenues to be gained through aggressive marketing, began, in the words of Lawrence Rubin, "to capitalize, if not prey, on deeply entrenched popular culture stereotypes." Those included the association of the tensions involved in everyday existence with a deterioration of brain function and the promise of curative action by the ingestion of prescribed capsules.[138]

Important also for our purposes was the implicit assumption that if a drug can resolve a mental problem, the condition of the given person had to be established as indicating an existing deficit. In contrast (thinking ahead to the ideas of Kierkegaard that we will discuss in Chapter 3), the inevitable tensions and bouts of depression that can be termed "problems in living" have most assuredly been experienced by schizophrenics and the depressed.[139] Their so-called difficulty, however, may often be the result of an honest and courageous confrontation with the real, as opposed to those who live in a denial, not uncommonly, a repressed or medicated denial, of the nature of their existential gloom and the level of their own psychic stability. Still, in the new economy of anxiety, blame, and fear of the outcast (with undisputed medical verification there to reinforce those determinations), perhaps the deepest irony and injustice of all is that many of the very ones with a truthful understanding of reality are frequently the target of punitive sanction.[140] Grant Gillet writes perceptively that one should therefore "expect the schizophrenic patient to be alienated from a world in which others feel secure and assured in their mental life and are cognitively supported by concurrence in judgment with others."[141]

The case of Ladaro Pennix is relevant in this regard. A politically active (prophetic) prisoner, his actions, which led to his transfer to a Special Housing Unit populated by the mentally ill, corroborate the way a determination to face day to day existence head on can be manipulated into a diagnosis of mental incompetence, with both the surrounding stigma and its retributive consequence. He was punished after urging his fellow detainees to recognize that their mental health is not the question and to resist being labeled, as he was, mentally deficient:

> Do not allow these officials to cower under the cloak of their bully tactics by making you keep your mouth shut … make you seem like an irrational compulsive adolescent or make you appear crazy. You are none of the above and you are actually smarter and more equipped to battle injustice than you realize.[142]

Of like interest is the case of Robert Richter. Equally adamant in his vocal revilement of the conditions which he and so many others are forced to endure, he wrote "to every address I could get" for four years. One of his missives was sent to a government official who promptly alerted the state police. Charged with trying to bribe a political figure, he was quickly sequestered in an Office of Mental Health strip cell for five days without food and then spent two months in solitary confinement. Upon completion of that ordeal, he was threatened again with the strip cell if he refused to take anti-psychotic drugs. He was told: "Cooperate with your treatment." Yet, he never received a diagnosis. In his commentary he states: "I was told that there was no diagnosis … It was Soviet style psychiatry: medicate away any new ideas people call crazy to hide the truth they speak."[143] Another "militant" prisoner came to the same conclusion: "If you try to stand together, they treat you with Thorazine."[144]

Angela Davis, in her account of incarceration in a New York City jail, testifies to the use of the drug to sedate otherwise healthy inmates who were consequently diagnosed as insane. Housed in the mental health unit rather than the general population, she recounts that upon entering the dayroom, the women gathered there "did not even notice that a new prisoner had been thrown in with them." They were "completely absorbed in themselves, blank stares telling me that no matter how much I wanted to talk, it would be futile to approach any of them. Later I learned that these women had received Thorazine with their meals each day, even if they were completely sane."[145]

Critics of Thorazine and other similar prophylactics point out that there is by no means consensus on how such remedies actually overcome the condition they were designed to address. As one study contends, "we still don't have anything like a theory of mental illness that is good enough to be wrong."[146] From Ian Evison's perspective, many psychiatrists have candidly acknowledged that "the high hopes for 'cures' to the major problematic states that accompanied the introduction of antipsychotic drugs in the late fifties were inflated." He points to the hordes of homeless on the streets, many of whom have been funneled in and out of the jail system, as a poignant reminder.[147]

Nevertheless, psychiatry has tethered itself to the ubiquitous reliance upon prescribed medications magnified in assertive marketing. For example, prescribed suppositories accounted for approximately 8 percent of the mental health budget in 1986; by 2009, that percentage had tripled.[148] For Alexander and Selesnick, the diagnostic issue has receded in favor of a "new conviction" that whatever may be its cause, "the disturbed mind can now be cured by drugs and that the patient himself as a person no longer needs to try to understand the source of his troubles."[149] Rubin expands this notion in asserting a flanking strategy necessary to uphold this pharmaceutical edifice, one of marginalization and decontextualization. As to the first, "marginalization involves simplifying the physician's role to that of a technician primed to dispense pills according to scripted cultural stereotypes." Regarding decontextualization, he refers to the "elimination of the personal, social, and cultural contexts of people's lives from the explanatory equation … entrenching the medicalization of non-medical problems."[150]

Whitaker's appraisal of the matter, not unlike that of Angela Davis, is disturbingly revelatory. He writes that the task of neuroleptics "is induce a *pathological* deficiency in dopamine transmission … 'a therapeutic Parkinsonism.'" This, in turn, has become not only "the standard fare in psychiatry," it has also become "the face of madness." What he means is that the very image of the schizophrenic "madman" is not schizophrenia in whatever might be its natural state. He then writes: "All of the traits that we have come to associate with schizophrenia—the awkward gait, the jerking arm movements, the vacant facial expression, the sleepiness, the lack of initiative—are symptoms due, at least in part, to a drug-induced deficiency in dopamine transmission."[151]

In his biting commentary of the "scientism" that dwarfs all but the standard procedures in biological psychiatry and neuroscience, including the default dependence upon medications, Raymond Tallis, also a neurologist, describes the ideology underlying such tactics as "neuromania," the adamant belief that consciousness is identical with neural activity.[152]

John Swinton, for this part, labels such reductionism as "pharmacomania." He shares the story of attending the lecture of a friend and medical colleague who surmised that he only needs 15 minutes with patients during which time he is looking, not at them, but "at the computer screen trying to sort out their meds."[153]

Drawing this section to a close, a 2008 study, mentioned by Harrington, reveals the cloudiness of both the prevailing medical judgment regarding disturbed patients and its arsenal of aggressive pills readily dispensed to combat their condition. She relates that when a group of researchers launched a multipart project designed to identify and critically assess all the relevant data established for schizophrenia, "seventy-seven candidate facts" were selected. Yet, "even the most robust individual facts pointed in a range of different directions" with no established consensus regarding the condition. As these researchers reflected in 2011, the conclusions reached by those at the forefront of the psychiatric profession seemed to be operating "like the fabled six blind Indian men groping different parts of an elephant and coming up with different conclusions."[154]

Still, one conclusion does *not* waver in the shifting terrain of the hyper-biological landscape of the contemporary psychiatric enterprise, it is revealed in the mantric deployment within the literature of physicians that regularly uses the term mental "disorder," rather than suspected illness, in discussions of questionable cerebral conditions.[155]

Diagnostic and Statistical Manual (DSM)

Now that intrusions into the body dominated the approach to mental illness, the psychiatric community turned its attention to diagnostics.[156] The result was the Diagnostic and Statistical Manual (DSM). It debuted in 1952, the first of five editions to this point. It has often been referred to as "the bible of psychiatry."[157] The way the resource is utilized is worthy of note, especially with the arrival of DSM-III when "personality disorders achieved widespread official recognition as a separate clinical diagnostic class of their own."[158] A technician surveys the written criteria for inclusion or exclusion of a particular behavioral category in the case of a specific individual. If the list of inclusive symptoms reaches a pre-determined tipping point, then it is safe to say, from the most advanced scientific standpoint, that the patient is inflicted with the malady.[159]

While the manual's various revisions have certainly involved greater procedural sophistication, it may come as no surprise that the most respected minds in the psychiatric community have faltered on perhaps the most fundamental question of all: what exactly constitutes the norm of sanity against which any determination of mental illness can be measured? De Young writes that "nowhere in any of the iterations of the *DSM* can a diagnosis of 'sane' be found or, for that matter, a description of it."[160] One finds a condition unidentified in one edition appearing in subsequent volumes, or a behavior classified as proof of cognitive incapacitation in one iteration disappearing completely in subsequent revisions. As to the former, the authors of one study relate that neither posttraumatic stress disorder nor borderline personality disorder were included in the manual's catalogue of illnesses until the publication of DSM-III in 1980. In like manner, acute stress disorder, bipolar II disorder, and Asperger's did not exist until they were introduced into DSM-IV in 1994.[161] This upswing in the enumeration of mental handicaps was the direct result of the expanding dominance of stringently biological determinations about which we have spoken. For example, in the original 1952 edition, 106 forms of mental illness were listed; DSM-II (1968) raised the number to 182; DSM-III (1980) itemized 285; and DSM-IV topped the list with 307.[162]

As to the disappearance of an ailment that was featured in earlier volumes, the case of homosexuality provides a telling example. Determined to be a sexual deviation in the first two editions, in the third, with the arrival of a new focus upon personality defects, it was categorized, under certain conditions, as a form of insanity. Yet, when the third edition was re-edited, the concept and its accompanying deleterious diagnosis entirely vanished.[163]

While the re-editing process in the matter just mentioned has saved much aggravation, not to mention (perhaps further) recrimination against the gay community, Louis Charland contends that the application of the mentally dis-functional label was not simply a *faux pas* but an instance of a wider problem: the failure to distinguish between socio-moral and medical conditions.[164] In fact, he states that the failure of the DSM to live up to its pledge of "fact and objectivity" is evident in that both the categories and criteria for verifying the presence of a problem requiring psychiatric intervention "are heavily evaluative." This criticism, he states, "has been ably defended from a variety of different points of view."[165] Another source observes that while DSM is the only conceptual framework psychiatry has, "it is widely believed to have flaws that run deep. The primary one is that its taxonomy of disease is based on the signs and symptoms of mental illness ... and not on the biological reality that grounds our understanding of physical disease."[166] Finally, in another report, the revisions already mentioned which saw a pronounced rise in designations of incapacity have met with widespread dissatisfaction as the criteria "do not sufficiently differentiate disorders ... diagnoses lack specificity for selection of treatment ... and many observed syndromes do not fit any diagnostic definition."[167]

The DSM has three classes of ailments, arranged in clusters. Cluster A targets "eccentric disorders" such as paranoia and schizophrenia; Cluster B involves those that are "dramatic or theatrical," the bearers of which are "asocial, histrionic, and narcissistic"; while those in Cluster C have "anxious and fearful disorders" and are obsessive compulsive, avoidant, and dependent.[168] One cryptic summation of the taxonomy that I have heard is: mad, bad, and sad. Yet, Charland contends that the abnormalities mentioned in Cluster B, for instance, are "not natural in any plausible sense," as they are heavily interactive and "too transient to count as genuine natural disease entities." As conditions in the life world change, so, too, "do the boundaries of deviant moral behavioral syndromes that are thought to require special social attention and behavioral control."[169]

Allow me to share an example of another prisoner acting from, what I perceive to be, a prophetic mandate, and summarily banished from his peers as "asocial, histrionic and narcissistic," to underscore the sorts of official determinations that shed light upon Charland's point. Willie Williams, imprisoned in Illinois, was placed in solitary confinement after internal intelligence read several letters indicating his dissatisfaction with what he contended were the inhumane conditions in his facility. Furthermore, he encouraged "political and legal minded inmates" to organize and seek amelioration both internally and with the aid of reform organizations. After prison authorities discussed his case, he was subsequently transferred out of general population and placed in solitary confinement. The justification for the maneuver was the accusation that he was a high-ranking member of a gang. Williams declares the speciousness of the charge but, more to the point, he reveals that the particular unit to which he was sent was coded "S.M.I, Severely Mentally Ill."[170]

Paula Caplan provides an explanation for the recognizable flaws in a resource often cast in biblical terms for its methodological refinement and unmatched intellectual acumen. She states that the entire classification of symptoms and diagnoses in the DSM is shielded by powerful gatekeepers who, she maintains, render anything but strictly scientific explanations for the decisions regarding "which diagnoses will be allowed through and which will be kept out of the handbook."[171] If her critique has substance, part of the reason may be explained by the fact that DSM-III was a worldwide best seller, generating massive profits for its publisher, the American Psychiatric Association.[172] Dr. Tom Insel, former head of the National Institute of Mental Health, would seem to sustain the contention that the aura of the DSM pales if one relies solely on the rigorousness of the science involved in its analytical results. He remarks that it has "100 percent reliability and 0 percent validity."[173]

Regardless of these charges and a slight diminution in its authoritative command, the DSM remains the resource most often relied upon by psychiatrists in determining who is truly "sick in the head," and, *a fortiori*, who goes to see her doctor or therapist and who spends the night in jail.[174]

Conclusion

We have spent a lot of time in this chapter on the evolution of the meaning of mental illness and how it has been perceived from religious, moral, therapeutic, and biological perspectives. We have witnessed the evolution of outlandish behavior beginning with its codification as a mystery revealing either angelic or demonic inspiration and, not infrequently, an aura of reverence in the case of personages such as Homer or Plato; one of heartfelt care witnessed in the practices of various Catholic religious orders; and, at least, one of respectful distance in recognition of its strange attunement to otherworldly powers.

That interpretive context honoring the innate interface of the material and the metaphysical was slowly and inexorably dismissed, beginning with the demise of the feudal enterprise and the wholesale release of the dispossessed and desperate who could not or would not be admitted into the new acquisitive economy. Those "masterless" men and women with their "fantasticall imaginacions" were herded by the thousands into workhouses and, most cogently, away from the affairs of the "sane" and well-to-do.

We then noted the attempts of some asylum managers to defend the ontological goodness of their patients and the psychic stability of most. Later, we looked briefly at two of the leading pioneers in the discipline of psychology, Freud and Jung, to embellish the primacy of the unconscious and its primordial, "essential," and determinative influence upon the psyche. Both approaches were largely dismissed as the medicalization of mental illness made its deliberate and, ultimately, complete sweep of competing explanations for those who are emotionally, cognitively, and spiritually different. This advance was accompanied, not without profound significance, by a return to the earlier post-feudal reaction to the dispossessed that resulted in an authoritative coloring of the "insane" with the brush of delinquency.

A medical designation of madness, and the "expert" opinion it demonstrates is the definitive and, for our purposes, the single most culpable factor in determining the sad fate of so many assessed as mentally impaired. Former Nobel Prize winning doctor, Eric Kandel, is among biology's most influential voices. He states: "As research into the brain and mind advances, it appears increasingly likely that there are actually no profound differences between neurological and psychiatric illnesses and that as we understand them better, more and more similarities will emerge."[175]

Roy Branson provides an explanation for the heady confidence of revered figures such as Dr. Kandel and the widespread appeal of somatic diagnoses and, not uncommonly, penal interventions in which so many of his colleagues have placed their trust: "It is understandable that medicine would achieve such an exalted status in American society; that it would be trusted not only to control but define deviancy. What could be more appropriate than a group so obviously dedicated to order and effectiveness deciding what constitutes deviance?"[176]

Scull's commentary is also worthy of note here. As he surveys the 200-year history of forcible confinement of those relegated to the margins of lucidity, what he calls a "history of reform without change," he supports the idea that those stalwart supporters of the psychiatric paradigm over that span of time have "sought to deflect attention away from the horrors of the present by resurrecting the tales of the barbarities of the past." In fact, he suggests that one of the discipline's primary ideological tasks "has been to manufacture reassurance of this sort, supplying us with a seemingly inexhaustible store of exemplary tales to document the inhumanities of earlier generations and the heroic struggles through which we arrived at our present (relative) state of grace and enlightenment."[177]

While the victory of biological analysis has been accomplished, there are cracks beginning to appear throughout the paradigm. Ones that serve, from the perspective of this book, to guide the reader to reconsider that many of those voices, subliminal messages, and unconscious motivations to utter sounds or perform gestures of protest are prophetic in nature. Yet the analysis proffered by specialists, despite scattered expressions of protest, brooks little or no dissent from the public at large and, perhaps more consequentially, from the judicial and penal sectors.[178] And it is that analysis that is, in many instances, the efficient cause that has washed the inhabitants of the rising reservoir of the crazed and unstable, overwhelmingly colored by their class, race, and their habitation on "the wrong side of the tracks," into their semi or permanent home behind the guard towers and barbed wire fences of our jails and prisons.

A prominent challenge to the Procrustean bed created by the reduction of brain function to a set of socially as well as medically prescribed functions is offered by the subfield of Neurodiversity within the discipline of Psychology. The authors of one study refer to the concept as an exploration of variations "in cognitive, affectual, and sensory functioning differing from the majority of the general population or … the 'neurotypical' population." They castigate the "medical, economic, and social interventions" that view subjects "as deviants" and victims of "internal and external oppression" due to myopic "standards of intellectual, perceptual, and emotional processing."[179]

Theological ethicists have their own set of coordinates to spurn bio-dominant analyses in favor of diverse approaches to moral reasoning. Sidney Callahan cautions that no "whole person" can be "reduced to his or her organic subsystems or be categorized as a set of symptoms of a disease." She contends, rather, that each human being is a synthesis of mind, body, and spirit that form a complex unity "energized by a vital healing life force that strives for health and wholeness."[180] William May probes the social and, ultimately punitive, psychology that is, in his view, overly determined by resistance to what is determined to be negative. He believes that "the ministrations of the professional" seed the fears that blossom into visceral public outcry and, of equal valence, the subconscious ethos of medical experts. Such primal opposition "usually imposes on others what it seeks to depose" and its reflexive reaction is most alarmingly evident in what he terms the "absolute negatives of madness, crime, dependency, and decrepitude." In a fitting summary of the argument thus far, he adds that when the curtailment of these conditions fails—as indeed they must, since the very hierarchy of money and power assure such "absolute negatives"—the persons so labeled "must be sequestered or eliminated by being sequestered."[181]

Some dissenting voices speak to us from the past. Karl Jaspers had a keen sense of the mysterious forces that lie in the depths of the patients with whom he worked and about whom he wrote. His remonstration against the biological model, whose dominance he both foresaw and with which he lived until his death, is as relevant now as it was a century ago. He observes the tendency "to discuss all psychic events as if their essence were something somatic, already in one's grasp." As a result of this deduction, "an imaginary 'soma' receives great emphasis as a heuristic presupposition, when in fact it is nothing but the unconscious expression of an unscientific prejudice."[182] In a more recent report, Joel and Ian Gold offer a rather humorous aphorism to orchestrate the same point. They write that the problem with the biological model is its overly broad generalizations regarding both the origin of "sickness" and the shape of its cure: "If its news to you … that real life tends to be messier than our idealizations, you are probably too young to drive."[183]

Having traced the development of mental illness in its various religious, classical, social, psychological, and medical incarnations, we now turn to the ideological underpinnings that have enabled the materialist reductionism of which we have just spoken to dominate the ethical, political, and economic discourse in the wider society as well as in the medical community. It is a discourse that has provided the authoritative sanction to allow biological determinism to control the prognosis and treatment of mental illness, identify its most socially toxic representatives, and watch as that massive number are then remanded to custodial isolation.

2

How We Think about
the Mentally Ill

In Chapter 1, we referred to a strategy of moral treatment of those sent to the asylums supervised by Philippe Pinel, Samuel Tuke, and William Connolly. This may sound presumptuous, but I am assuming that the designation did not elicit pause, let alone discomfort, among some readers. And the very fact that it may not have is why it is important at this juncture to suggest that among the serious issues that confront us in discussing "loaded" terms such as the morality of the understanding of and response to those who think and act irregularly, the metaethical question, or what Kant calls transcendental philosophy, is, I believe, at the forefront.[1]

Thus, in this chapter, I want to emphasize why our focus is not on which of the two approaches we have looked at is more ethical than its counterpart. Everyone involved in this, or any other matter of personal choice or public policy, is doing exactly what they consider to be proper given their foundational, pre-reflexive starting points from which they frame pertinent moral issues and the particular circumstances relative to them. The real question is language: how we talk about people, who and what they are by nature, and what they are capable of being and doing. It will, therefore, be our present focus to try to uncover the implicit assumptions within the two ways of perceiving suspected insanity spoken of in the last chapter, not to question the personal integrity of people on either side of the issue. I have tried to show that no specific person or structural regimen is patently right or wrong (the history of the treatment of those reputed to be mentally ill reveals many sad tales, regardless of the time period); but there are radically distinct foundational principles and ethical premises in the different methodologies that have virtually everything to do with the approaches that we have discussed thus far. The first is driven by a belief that might be termed incarnational: the physical and metaphysical have their own irreducible integrity and, moreover, are mutually interdependent; the second is predicated upon a materialist and behaviorist hypothesis that evaluates sense experience and biological function as fully constitutive of the given person's psyche and, consequently, denies the existence of ideas or phenomena outside the realm of the data provided by such quantifiable knowledge.

While I wish to avoid dualist reductionism or a crude zero sum equation, the argument that follows is predicated upon a porous relationship between the material and the metaphysical as found in perennial religious thought and its philosophical and therapeutic accompanists. It is an anthropology that magnifies the role of direct experience of the unseen and the intuitive in inspiring (prophetic) protest against violence generally and violence against the poor and vulnerable in particular. Having stated that ideological preference, we will now investigate the worldviews about which we have spoken.

Ethics, language, and human nature

Returning to the mention of moral treatment, there is a thinly hidden assumption in the term implying that the way previous administrators (upon whom both Pinel and Tuke, particularly, poured caustic disfavor) or, for that matter, later superintendents who turned increasingly toward strictly medical prognoses and physical remedies were unethical or, at least, delinquent in their ethical development. That is a facile comparison that is, I believe, inappropriate to our task to "think" those defined as abnormal not only out of the penal facilities where large numbers are forced to dwell, but also out of the conceptual prisons that are the real locus of our anxieties about and disregard for so many in this population. The true source of the conflict, then and now (here remembering Suzanne Langer's work) is an ethical horizon so embedded, so ingrained, and so "second skin like" that we rarely stop to ponder that others see the world and form their ethical deductions just as automatically from a fundamentally different horizon: one's "ways of thinking ... are not avowed by the average [person], but simply followed. He is not conscious of assuming any basic principles. They are what a German would call his 'Weltanschauung' ... They constitute his outlook; they are deeper than facts he may note or propositions he may moot."[2] Wittgenstein says of this cognitive realm: "I cannot touch it."[3] Or, one might rearrange the epigram of Alasdair MacIntyre. The question is not which of the two approaches to mental illness is moral, but whose morality and which rationality?[4]

Another way to pose the metaethical question is through the concept of neurodiversity about which we spoke in the last chapter. Humans process input from both the phenomenal and the noumenal in different ways. While there are, indeed, privileged epistemologies, there is no correct way, according to proponents, to conceptualize another's experiential reservoir and the conclusions that proceed effortlessly from it.[5] That said, day to day to practice and policy lag far behind the level of tolerance and appreciation of psychic difference that the theory calls for.

In his play, *Six Characters in Search of an Author*, Nobel laureate, Luigi Pirandello, gives poetic voice to the way an imperial and single-minded neurological perspective easily creates reflexive patterns that are both parochial and reductionist upon encountering the "other." He writes that

> each of us thinks of himself as *one* but that, well, it's not true, each of us is many, oh so many, sir, according to the possibilities of being that are in us. We are one thing for this person, another for that! Already *two* utterly different things! ... It's not true! Not true! We realize as much when, by some unfortunate chance, in one or another of our acts, we find ourselves suspended, hooked. We see, I mean, that we are not wholly in that act, and therefore that it would be abominably unjust to judge us by that act alone, to hold us suspended, hooked, in the pillory, our whole life long, as if our life was summed up in that act![6]

Pirandello is thus reaffirming in poignant terms that it is best to acknowledge that there is indeed a massive divide in the way the "taken for granted" is understood in the two neurological and ethical outlooks we are analyzing. The divide is not ultimately unbridgeable, but it serves no purpose to denigrate people for the way reality appears to them and the, sometimes, virulent responses that arise when their unshakable world construct is destabilized. Everything turns on the entrenched assumptions of the debate about who is crazy, why or why not they are crazy, and what procedural steps are essential either to isolate the sick ones or, perhaps, attend to the truths they communicate.

Since I am engaging in cautionary preliminaries, allow me to repeat once more that mental illness is not a fabrication. There are many with both organic handicaps as well as neurotic phobias, delusions, and psychotic projections who are deeply dangerous to themselves and those around them. Such persons can and do benefit from the abundant resources of the therapeutic and psychiatric professions. The principal focus of the ensuing pages is not the *explicit* justifications utilized to expunge an overwhelming number of men and women whose inner instinctual and imaginative experience is, to them, not only noetic but also compelling and authoritative (referring here to our focus on the prophetic); that was our task in the last chapter. Rather, our intention now is to disclose what I perceive to be the covert and subliminal (metaethical) assumptions that, remembering Pirandello, suspend and hook others in the pillory their whole life long. It is these subliminal intimations that provide the nourishment for those social, legal, and medical determinations.

We will proceed now to survey each of the ideological starting points.

Ethical universalism, a-historicity, and its response to the (presumably) mentally ill

I have to say that, as a professor, I have grown so weary of trying to change student language regarding ethics that, often, I allow casual statements such as so and so "lacks a moral compass," or what he or she did was "totally unethical" go unchallenged. That strategy is not only pragmatic, as it tends to derail conversation, but is also largely an affirmation that objections to patterned linguistic expressions tend to be self-defeating as such clichés are part and parcel of the day to day syntax of most value-laden conversations that most people, not only students, engage in. Of course, that is the reality of the *weltanschauung* about which Langer speaks.

To say that such day to day to grammar is significant is an understatement. Like our rather brief inquiry into psychiatric history, I will not tax the reader's patience or knowledge with a detailed analysis of the assumptions hidden in quotidian discourse. I do want, however, to suggest that the dream of Enlightenment thinkers, however postmodern we may be, to escape the destructive polemics of religious bickering by locating the roots of ethics in strict scientific procedure and anatomical function (Hobbes, Francis Bacon, and others), or in a universal, rational, categorical imperative (Kant and deontological ethics), or in calculating the costs and benefits of a given course action with only pleasure and pain as the constant mediators of the equation (Bentham, Mill, and the tradition they initiated), or in universal moral sentiments (David Hume, Thomas Hutchison, Adam Smith, and those who honor moral sense theory), has set the limits of contemporary "true discourse" and its moral commitments and assumptions.[7]

While the first of these (scientific deduction) normally lacks any specifically stated ethical directives, save the procedural guidelines necessary to ensure that proven theories are properly duplicated, the latter three, despite the differences between them, all build upon subjective foundations: each person possesses within him or herself the capacity to know and perform normative moral requirements. In each, a rational, "disengaged" being, what Charles Taylor has labeled the "punctual self," seeks to gain some functional control of a disenchanted world shorn of classical philosophical and theological beliefs in which the individual was called upon to tailor her ethical choices in conformity to truths that transcend personal feeling and cognitive calculation.[8]

I have argued in another context, borrowing an idea from John Milbank, that all the ethical theories that provide the values implicit in our linguistic constructions (however deeply divided and rancorous they may often be) have one thing in common. Each requires, at some terminal point, the need to exercise violent intervention to corral, re-educate, or punish those who fail to adhere to the commonly available and obligatory rational directives, or whose hedonic calculus instigates actions harmful to what the majority have determined to be the greatest good, or whose application of the sentiments that inform human action spurns the moderation called for by the internal "impartial spectator."[9]

Such forceful intervention, as we have seen, was, for the most part, the only means available in a world left without the normative guideposts that certain religious and ethical traditions had upheld such as (in an ideal typical sense) the obligation to care for the poor and vulnerable and the means to overcome human error by means of penance, rather than through coercion. A case in point from a legal and penal perspective, one most relevant to our study of the persecution of the prophetic, is provided by former Yale law professor, Robert Cover. He writes that criminal jurisprudence "is either played out on the field of pain and death or it is something less (or more) than law."[10] "[J]udges deal pain and death. That is not all that they do ... But they do deal pain and death. From John Winthrop to Warren Burger they have sat atop a pyramid of violence."[11] In his words, the "jurispathic profession" is constrained by the positivist moral language that dominates legal thought. Its ahistorical disinterest in the multiplicity of religious and cultural practices, and its emphasis simply upon the law as written, leaves no room for appreciation of other ways of knowing and practicing the right and the good, only for the abject use of force to elicit compliance. He notes that such "logic" is evoked when judges "confronting the luxuriant growth of a hundred legal traditions" rule "that this *one* is law and destroy or try to destroy the rest."[12]

Weber comes to a similar conclusion in his commentary on "The Sermon on the Mount" and its injunction to "offer no resistance" to the evildoer (Mt. 5:39). Such pious phrases are anathema to the state credo which avows: "You shall have the right to triumph by the use of force, otherwise you too may be responsible for injustice." In fact, Weber insists that without such violent incursion, the state could not exist since, in the final analysis, it "depends ultimately upon power relations and not on 'ethical right'."[13]

Langer argues that wedding procedures of thought (what Kant called "appearance") with strict scientifically sanctioned empiricism, including its statutory, penal, and medical derivatives, inevitably yields a positivist offspring.[14] It is manifested, as we will see, in "an appeal to common-sense against the difficulties of establishing metaphysical or logical 'first principles' ... [It] entertains no ... doubts, and raises no epistemological problems; its belief in the veracity of sense is implicit and dogmatic."[15]

From the perspective of Theodor Adorno, the logic of the various (liberal) philosophical perspectives that have been mentioned, with their focus on interiority and the desire "to eliminate the traditional moments of thinking" seeks, as Cover maintains, to "dehistoricize the contents of thought and assign to history a special, fact-gathering branch of science ...

The fictitious one-dimensional Now became the cognitive ground of all inner meaning."[16] Put another way, Adorno argues that since the sciences made their "irrevocable farewell to idealistic philosophy," they established their legitimacy solely on the basis of the method employed to determine the hypothetical meaning of a specific area of study or, in our case, a specific human being. This "self-exegesis makes a *causa sui* of science. It accepts itself as given and thereby sanctions also its currently existing form." Thus, he maintains, with its "ideal of positivity," the sciences, particularly the intellectual ones, "lapse into the irrelevance and nonconeptuality of countless special investigations."[17]

Adorno, as many know, is just as opposed to beliefs in ontologically grounded first principles as he is in current, a-historical forms of knowledge wherein the acting subject, as previously mentioned, assumes a privileged interpretive position vis-à-vis the world around him or her.[18] Still, he echoes Taylor's notion of the "punctual self," a person who makes immediate assumptions about the "now," the truth of which grounds sufficiently and, often, irrevocably the meaning of the event or the person performing it.

It is at this stage that the thought of Nietzsche is so important in our exposition. In seeking to trace the origins of an epistemology and ethics based upon the dismissal of the spiritual in favor of the material, he points out that the casualty in this transformation was not only Christianity, despite all of its well-orchestrated flaws (that he made no attempt to conceal), but also the worldview of lyric poetry, in which the self was seen to dwell "truly and eternally, in the ground of being."[19]

The new ethos and anthropology were birthed in the Age of Reason— at the very time when the confinement of the "mad" became both customary and obligatory.[20] As a result, the conceptual "ground of being," the understanding of the person, and the religious origins of good and evil, were discarded in favor of a portrait of value and worth painted in terms of the "responsibility" one owes to one's betters (their betterment defined in terms of their ability to create "sane" and meticulously binding measures of expectation and performance). It is a view of the individual that owes its origin, in Nietzsche's words, to a "secret, malicious desire to belittle humanity" out of "resentment of Christianity." It defines personal experience and its meaning exclusively in terms of a "social straight jacket" whose lining is sewn with an evaluation of all creaturely endeavor in terms of number, degree, size, and shape. It accomplished the feat of turning each person into a being who is now fully "regular, uniform ... calculable." This dramatic recreation of the epicenter of meaning "constitutes the long history of the origins of *responsibility*." It is likened to the "particular task of breeding an animal with the prerogative to promise" and includes "the more immediate task of first *making* man to a certain degree necessary, uniform, a peer amongst peers, orderly and consequently predictable."[21]

In this, Nietzsche further contends—hearkening back to the subjective interiority in "modernist" theories—that in this dramatic anthropological turn both society and morality "finally reveal what they were," that is to say, "simply *the means to*." Thus, "we then find the *sovereign individual* as the ripest fruit on its tree, like only to itself, having freed itself from the morality of custom, an autonomous, supra-ethical individual."[22]

Foucault, who in demonstrative ways assumed the Nietzschean mantle, summarizes the former's insight into a new *episteme*, literally the "birth of man." He states that "no philosophy, no political or moral option, no empirical science of any kind, no observation of the human body, no analysis of sensation, imagination, or the passions, had ever encountered, in the seventeenth or eighteenth century, anything like man." Indeed, for he and Nietzsche, the evaluative measure of personhood lodged within the linguistic patterns of current conversation was unknown until that time; and it was precisely at that juncture that the human sciences made their appearance and "it was decided to include man ... among the objects of science."[23]

Again, channeling Nietzsche, Foucault writes that the new basis of truth extends "the principle and movement of a human destiny to even the smallest particles of nature." All things available to sensual perception were drawn into the same evaluative and politically charged current.[24]

This striking alteration was manifested in the birth of behaviorism: a fully materialist reduction of the human to the union of Lockean empiricism and utilitarian pleasure/pain calculation. We saw the former in the transformation of the asylum into a domain in which complete environmental control was the only admissible explanation for the dysfunctional antics of the patients exemplified in the techniques manufactured by a noteworthy heir to Locke's empiricism, Benjamin Rush.

Behaviorism has, in many ways, become the coin of the realm in the sciences; its postulates used to justify not only the strictly biological approach to those patients selected for medical intervention, but also that of the social sciences, generally, and criminology in particular. An author whose work has been most influential in this regard is B.F. Skinner. We will see his hand in the reformulation of the concept of rehabilitation as an adjunct to aggressive forms of social control; and it cannot be denied that a behaviorist strategy, so dependent on the Lockean belief of the mind as an "empty cabinet" prone for aggressive re-socialization, has helped to underwrite the massive rise in penal commitments.

Skinner writes that objectionable behavior, in whatever guise the positivist canon frames it, cannot be addressed successfully save by the aid of "reinforcers" to stimulate the psyche into obedience:

> The real issue is the effectiveness of techniques of control. We shall not solve problems of alcoholism and juvenile delinquency by increasing

a sense of responsibility. It is the environment which is "responsible" for the objectionable behavior, and it is the environment, not some attribute to the individual, which must be changed.[25]

Here we have the perfect contemporary example of the commitment to render human conduct malleable to the architects of order and norm, those before whom, in Nietzschean parlance, those without power must prostrate themselves. Skinner states that science provides an explanation of human behavior whose task is "the destruction of mystery." In such a schema, some form of punishment becomes the only recognizable mode "to induce people *not* to behave in given ways."[26]

Behaviorism is ubiquitous in criminological literature. In the words of one study: "Correctional programming in many ways is no different from medical, psychiatric or substance abuse treatment. These formal interventions by nature are symptom-focused, and therefore, deficit-based. Ameliorate the symptom and the disease process is contained and managed, if not eliminated."[27] D.A. Andrews and James Bonta build their influential theory of rehabilitative intervention, in part, upon "the radical behaviorism of Skinner."[28]

William James, in his study of religious experience, was keen to point out both the pitfalls and growing influence of a dogma bent upon destroying mystery. He prefigured the triumph of biological explanations and therapeutics regarding the mentally ill in his barbed commentary on what he termed "medical materialism": the reduction of all phenomena to strictly organic explanation. In his mind, such a stance is driven far less by scientific precision than by a prejudicial animus, a *weltanschauung*, that seeks to discredit "states of mind for which we have an antipathy."[29]

Part and parcel of the worldview we are investigating, remembering Martin Buber, is the centrality of the "I-It" as opposed to the "I-Thou" relationship.[30] R.D. Laing employs this dyad in his analysis of contemporary psychiatry. He declares, in line with our emphasis on metaethics, that what he observes to be the "most serious objection to the technical vocabulary currently used to describe psychiatric patients is that it consists of words which split [the person] up verbally."[31] Elemental to this tactic is the division between a human being and an organism exhibiting a troubling symptom.[32]

In this, I am reminded of Paulo Freire's *Pedagogy of the Oppressed* wherein authentic communication and effective learning is impossible without a humble recognition of the dignity of the other:

> How can I dialogue if I regard myself as a case apart from others—mere "its" in whom I cannot recognize other "I's"? How can I dialogue if I consider myself … the owner of truth and knowledge …? How can I dialogue if I am closed to—and even offended by—the contributions of others?[33]

Hegel reacts similarly in his critique of the inbred tendency of science to turn phenomena and people into predicates: "Such predicates can be multiplied to infinity" as each determination can be used to sublimate other forms. "In this sort of circle of reciprocity one never learns what the thing itself is, nor what the one or the other is."[34]

For Vico, this official linguistic and political ethos that separates existence and essence forefronts the individual (remembering Pirandello) as she appears as opposed to the person that she is. It is an exemplar of the "Age of Men," a time of "limited ideas" featuring those who "have little capacity to understand the universal and eternal." The social yield of this epoch will be a people who are "barbaric and ferocious, for these are indivisible properties of such a nature."[35]

Vico thus anticipates Nietzsche in asserting that the aristocratic Age of Heroes, the predecessor of the Age of Men, was peaceable "as long as nobles kept the multitude satisfied with it." When, however, the nobles changed "from being magnanimous to cruel, they became so many minor tyrants." The ensuing "free" republics created legislative assemblies in which heroism became associated with democracy "in which free peoples exercise a mind empty of feeling" and find their enjoyment and retributive muscle in the law.[36]

As the foregoing exemplifies, an exaggerated dualism is an inevitable component of the perspective under question as it necessarily proceeds from impersonal calculation.[37] There can be no other world than the one based on the inherent division between the knower and what is known, the signifier and the signified (the "sane" determining who is "insane," for instance), since the primacy of subjective sense experience serves the habits of thought and consequent theories, not to mention the fears, fantasies, and projections of a largely unimpeachable moral source. Here, "the bourgeois *ratio*" can establish the comprehensive order within that it's positivist determinations have negated outside itself.[38] It represents "a new outlook on life," a "Cartesian age" of radical skepticism led by "a revolutionary generative idea: the dichotomy of all reality into *inner experience and outer world*, subject and object, private reality and public truth."[39] For Nietzsche's teacher, Schopenhauer, this overarching binary state of affairs is so solid a basis for its conclusions that "a reduction to this … can leave nothing to be desired."[40]

MacIntyre maintains that such a pronounced dualist methodology cannot avoid falling into the chasm of emotivism: that the meaning of any event is supplied solely by the independent internal judge whose application of reason, or whose pleasure/pain calculations, or whose employment of the moral sense is as inveterately ephemeral—given the frequent and, often, sudden changes in one's mental and emotional state—as it is certain of the veracity of its determinations. Worse, at least from MacIntyre's point of view, "to a large degree people now think, talk, and act *as if* emotivism were true … It has become embedded in our culture."[41] Thus, the very attempt to relativize all but the internal order, as the emotivist is bound to do, yields no order at all, only an "insatiable" will with few, if any, barriers to omnipotence.[42] For such a voracious will, of no small consequence for our purposes, what differs dramatically "from the existent will strike the existent as witchcraft."[43]

We have already suggested how such a primary ethical stance inevitably tumbles down the slope into a default imposition of violence. For within its principled contours, the state, with its complete and hyper-active monopoly over the use of force, is the final mediator of the endless claims to a proper resolution of conflicts between the uncontestable demands of rival autonomous wills. This is evidenced in a litigious culture and, anecdotally, in the ever-popular courtroom dramas that fill so much of afternoon programming, as well as in the real life and death dramas involving the mentally suspect and lethal state power.

A journalist who was investigating the shooting death of a person categorized as "deranged" describes how, when called to the scene, the officer labeled the victim as a "troublesome criminal." When asked to expand upon his thought pattern, he stated: "[W]hat crossed my mind was finding the bad guy." The officer was acting upon a dualist framework, a cultural stereotype of a world populated by the "good" and the "bad," and by distressing extension, between a mentally unorthodox person and a hoodlum.[44]

Other incidents paralleling this reductionist and oppositional worldview, with the same hyper-defensive and violent reaction, unfortunately abound. In a case from 2014, Kajieme Powell, who was "clearly mentally distraught and had a knife," took a few steps toward officers who were "dozens of feet away." Yet, rather than employ a more dialogical or, in any event, peaceful tactic, "they shot him to death."[45] A year later, the mother of Jason Harrison summoned assistance for her son who had refused to take his prescribed medication. When the squad car arrived, she went to meet the officer with Jason, who was carrying a screwdriver. Upon seeing him, the officer commanded him to drop the implement and, seconds later, shot and killed him.[46] Terse comments from a family member of the slain emoted: "[T]hey didn't have to shoot him like the way they killed him: like a … dog."[47]

Finally, in March 2020, at a time of widespread national protests in the US over the killing of black men by law enforcement officials, Daniel Prude ran almost naked out of his brother's home in Rochester, NY. His brother followed the customary social practice and called the emergency number—911. Several hours later, the police located him. The officers handcuffed him while another lodged his knee on Prude's back for several minutes. Unable to breathe, Prude lost consciousness and passed away a week later.[48]

To bring some statistical heft to these sad revelations, according to the Treatment Advocacy Center, one in every four killings made by police in the United States involves a person designated as mentally unstable; in fact, one so classified is 16 times more likely to be killed during an incident involving constabularies.[49]

It is important to remember, even in a chapter on theological and philosophical matters, that a theory only has validity if it is a truthful summary of a wealth of real-life experience and, all too often regarding the population we are studying, heart-rending experience.

To conclude this section: we have provided a short outline of the metaethical foundation of many of the policy decisions that have been made regarding the cerebrally suspect, particularly since the inception of their enforced institutionalization. Barring a broader evaluative component in the accumulation of sense impressions with which the actions of a particular person are weighed, the various quantifiable categories to which Nietzsche alludes serve to provide the substance from which judgments are formed, not only regarding the particular mental condition or pathology of a given patient, but also whether he or she is fit to live in consort with the rest of society or, in some cases, whether he or she is fit to live at all. No one is evil by nature; no one lacks a "moral compass" or is "unethical." There are, however, patently different moralities and rationalities. Perhaps this pithy aphorism from Hobbes is an appropriate summary of the all too real consequences of the disparity in worldviews: "Prophets can't be trusted."[50]

The permeable boundary between the physical and the metaphysical

I have insisted in the foregoing presentation that a materialist, a-historical perspective, regardless of the (presumed) good will of its proponents, lacks the categories, vocabulary, and presuppositions to appreciate, let alone adequately converse with, people whose actual experiences are patterned upon a deep mythic structure (here recalling Jung's archetypal arsenal). In the latter case, we speak of a world, timeless in the breadth of its grasp, that has provided the symbolic network to record and interpret the kinds of experiences that mystics, seers, and prophets claim to have had down through the ages.[51]

An illustration of this mode of being that would render one agape who is working from a rigorously empirical epistemology is recorded by Kent Nerbern. As he stood in a rocky creek bed in the remote wilderness of northern Alaska, Nerbern relates that those very stones suddenly began to speak:

> It was a clacking sound, a clattering sound, like the fluttering of wings, the descent of birds, the pounding of a hundred thousand hooves across the frozen tundra. I could not name it, but neither could I deny it. It came to me through senses unfamiliar, claiming me with a knowledge I did not know. That it was not within my rational understanding did not make it any less real.[52]

One might here recall the taxonomy of mystical experience offered by William James. In it, one is seized by an "ineffable" encounter in which one is "passive." Though it is short or "transient" in duration, the event always contains something "noetic."[53] As the reader is aware, the methodology that James adopts in *The Varieties of Religious Experience* is to present a formidable parade of "hysterics" who are, in his mind, the people who have done the most to change the world for the better.[54] His subjects were overcome by "nervous instability," "subject to abnormal psychical visitations," and all were "geniuses." The single most consistent qualification for both causes and effects is that for each "religion exists not as a dull habit, but as an acute fever." Despite "a discordant inner life," in which "frequently they have fallen into trances, heard voices, seen visions," such persons "have known no measure."[55]

Putting this Jamesean framework into theological terminology, Wolfhart Pannenberg states that imagination renders the person as both creative and yet dependent upon a deeper source of inspiration. Thus, he says that it is not without reason that "we speak of 'unexpected flights' of imagination." Yet, one cannot induce such revelations on her own. Rather, only in "a state of relaxation do images appear to 'flood' the imagination ... It is worth noting that individuals who are especially creative intellectually have emphasized the inspirational aspect of their insights."[56]

Hegel develops a sartorial metaphor to express the same point. He states that the "common road" of scientific empiricism "can be taken in casual dress." However, those who have a "high sense of the Eternal, the Holy, the infinite" make their way "in the robes of the high priest, on a road that is no road, but has immediate being as its centre, the genius of profound original ideas and lofty flashes of inspiration."[57]

This sudden creative impulse is exemplified in James' portrait of George Fox, the founder of the Quaker religion. James states that there can be "no better of example" of a "genius" of "unsound" mind, "a psychopath ... of the deepest dye," than Fox. The latter underwent a life-changing spiritual encounter as he and some associates were walking on a snowy afternoon near the town of Lichfield. As soon as he was apprised of the name of the town, Fox felt the sudden infusion of divine energy and appointment:

> I was commanded by the Lord to pull off my shoes. I stood still, for it was winter; but the word of the Lord was like a fire in me. So I put off my shoes and left them with the shepherds; and the poor shepherds trembled, and were astonished.

He then proceeded into the town when the word of God came to him again, commanding him to cry: "'Wo to the bloody city of Lichfield!' So I went up and down the streets, crying with a loud voice, Wo to the bloody city of Lichfield!" He then states that as he continued to cry, "there seemed to me to be a channel of blood running down the streets, and the market-place appeared like a pool of blood."[58] Later, Fox learned that in that very city a large number of Christians had been martyred long ago and it was his commission from God to speak on behalf of the memory of those fallen believers.

In keeping with our theme of the punishment of outlandish behavior and prophetic actions and insights, it is worth noting that the revelations Fox claims to have received from God also led him to decry all forms of violence, including military service, and any form of forced tithing or taxation. For his unorthodox views he was imprisoned eight times. In answer to his critics and, seemingly, the charge that he was out of his mind, he spoke on behalf of himself and his Quaker congregants, many of whom also suffered the pains of confinement:

> We are not furious, foolish, mad; but through patience and meekness have borne lies and slanders ... and have undergone great sufferings ... The spiritual [person] in not mad, foolish, furious ... but all are if a mad, foolish, furious spirit ... wrestles with flesh and blood with carnal weapons.[59]

These examples provide concrete instances of the fact that over the course of history, countless people, what can be termed "a neurominority," profess to have had such mystical experiences—direct contact with God, or some spiritual entity, that provides compelling glimpses into the meaning of reality that are so far from common sense logic and empirical documentation that they must either be honored, or dismissed, or perhaps punished as indisputable evidence of an individual who is "hysterical" and "psychopathic."[60] From this latter opinion, here quoting Fox, persons or policies that seek to wrestle "with flesh and blood with carnal weapons," as opposed to weapons of the Spirit, will label, stigmatize, forcibly intervene, and on many occasions violently treat those whose message is offensive and disconcerting to their confident intellectual assertions.

A current prisoner gives evidence to this in his disclosure that the practice of meditation has produced in him a degree of "militancy," perhaps not as confrontational as Fox or others to whom we have been introduced thus far, but still his daily devotion has led him to "look at life through 'signs' and 'cycles of energy.'" He states further that "a lot of people don't see what I see. I'm left to navigate through a lot of mental arrested developments" and ponder the many "martyrs of religion."[61]

This approach, which affirms that the boundary between the seen and unseen, between the empirical and what Kant calls the pure a-priori of the metaphysical, is penetrable and fluid, is what I want to further elucidate in this section.[62]

Continuing with Kant, his project in the *Critique of Pure Reason* was precisely to seek to understand by rational means, not only the reality, but also the necessity of the pure a-priori. As to its reality, he states that it is in the realm of knowledge beyond the senses "that our reason carries on those inquiries which owing to their importance we consider to be far more excellent, and in their purpose far more lofty, than all that the understanding can learn in the field of appearances."[63] And regarding its necessity, he states that "metaphysics actually exists, if not as a science, yet still as a natural disposition. For human reason ... proceeds impetuously, driven on by an inward need, to questions such as cannot be answered by any empirical employment of reason."[64]

Jaspers corroborates this innate longing for hidden or symbolic truths that provide comprehensive meaning to all that we absorb through the senses; an edifice of significance that Harvey Cox would later image as a "sacred canopy."[65] Jaspers contrasts two states of consciousness: the metaphysical and the psychological. The former "reaches after a meaning into which all other limited meanings can be taken up and absorbed." It is the "language of unconditioned being" lodged in the "soul" or "psyche" that is oriented to embrace the "fathomless meaning" inherent in all of reality.[66] He uses the metaphor of the ocean to describe the distinction between each viewpoint. He likens psychological conclusions regarding direct "psychic experiences" with the "foam on the sea's surface." It is unaware of the profound "depths" of the metaphysical which are inaccessible to it for such phenomena "can only be explored in an indirect and theoretical way."[67]

As for our focus on the proper way to approach the uncommon perceptions of the psychiatric patient, Jaspers continues that a human being cannot be reduced to "empirical reality" but bears a meaning that "we cannot verify." More to the point, this inherent sacredness "is not a matter for the science of psychopathology." Certainly, the medical and therapeutic professional "can help in clarifying the facts that will refine the experience" of understanding. However, those who manifest "psychotic states," thinking perhaps here of George Fox, also offer us "a human parable" in their sometimes "inverted and distorted attempts" to elaborate significant moral and spiritual issues that are "common to us all." It is the proper, yet, he thinks, largely unrealized task of the psychiatrist to see beyond what appear to be cognitive disorders in clients and into "depths which do not so much belong to their *illness* as to themselves as individuals with their own historical truth."[68] John Swinton echoes Jaspers in his contention that the inner life and integrity of persons diagnosed with severe cognitive malfunction are in no way prohibitive of unfathomable "spiritual experience and the development of authentic faith."[69]

A vivid example of the "historical truth" within the depths of a given soul fully outside of and, indeed, unknowable to a materialist epistemology is the occurrence of the "dark night." This is a pregnant metaphor in spiritual literature utilized by the sixteenth-century Spanish mystic, St. John of the Cross, in the poetry he wrote in his own time in captivity; his captors, no doubt, convinced of *his* madness. He alluded to the barrenness, loneliness, and anguish that the soul endures at certain times of life when all consolation and sense of the divine have evaporated and one must proceed in darkness (here paraphrasing) with no other light than that which burns in the heart.[70] We will come back to this inner state of desolation as we look in the coming chapters at the psychological and spiritual rudiments of the inner world that are at once so real and powerful to the recipients (among whom I include many of the prophets about whom we speak) and so strange and offensive to others, often, others with the power to subject them to punitive restraint.

Of the dark night experience, John writes that a "deeper enlightenment and wider experience than mine is necessary to explain the dark night through which a soul journeys toward that divine light of perfect union with God." In fact, the spiritual and temporal trials that must be endured "are so numerous and profound that human science cannot understand them adequately. Nor does experience of them equip one to explain them. Only those who suffer them will know what this experience is like, but they won't be able to describe it."[71]

Like many of the poor deposited in coercive quarantine per judicial and medical order, and in John's case, by his religious brethren, he also heard voices or what he terms "interior words." He calls such sounds "substantial" in that "they are impressed upon the soul in a definitely formal way." They "produce vivid and substantial effects upon the soul, whereas words which are merely formal do not."[72]

Complementing this in his own style, Schopenhauer writes that the intellectual sciences can reveal brute facts but are incapable of teaching us the meaning of phenomena: their "inner nature," their "natural force" which constitute and remain "an eternal secret."[73] He also honors, with different terminology, the knowledge that the unconscious reveals and its relation to what Jung calls archetypal symbolism. He writes that the contention that visionary dreams lack the "vividness and distinctness" of "real perception" is "not worth considering at all." Moreover, he uses the concept of "Maya" in the Hindu *Vedas* and *Puranas* to reveal that the "whole knowledge of the actual world," without the insight provided by the wisdom of the gods, is best interpreted as a dream.[74]

These accounts and explanations concerning a river of connection flowing through all cosmic elements, seen and unseen, suggest the rich concept of coherence. Whitehead uses that term liberally in positing the integral relation between all things in which "no entity can be conceived in complete abstraction from the system of the universe."[75] As a result, he maintains that it is the task of philosophy to challenge what he considers to be "the half-truths" that constitute scientific first principles: "All general truths condition each other; and the limits of their application cannot be adequately defined apart from their correlation by yet wider generalities."[76]

Whitehead's notion of coherence is most suitable to depict the notion of faith, intuitive knowing, and the concept of prophecy as we are employing it in this context. We will look more in depth at the latter in Chapter 4, but its relation to faith is paramount and, for both, a guiding proposition is that there is not only a deep pool of meaning in the world beyond the corporeal, but it also communicates a message of mutual indwelling and participation.

That is to say that faith is a dynamic and inclusionary stance in relation to life, all of life. In this it varies substantially from a concept often associated erroneously with it: belief. The latter concerns itself in asserting the truth of certain dogmatic propositions. A belief is a certitude; something about which one entertains no serious doubt. Faith, on the other hand, points to an opening of the mind and heart. It is a conviction that somehow God is present in a life-giving and life-affirming way in every moment one encounters, even, or perhaps especially, in the daily inner and outer turmoil, the "dark nights," faced by so many. Richard Rohr claims that such an opening to the intense beauty and pathos of life is necessary to help one move to new levels of consciousness. Faith does not concern itself with whether certain dogmas or moral positions are true but with a confidence that in each moment and in each encounter "Ultimate Reality/God/Jesus is accessible to us—and ... on our side."[77]

Rohr echoes Whitehead in maintaining that the very essence of faith is coherence, a common inner connectedness, a co-inheritance of grace and unconditioned divine favor that is universal and reaches all things, both material and immaterial. It is fully non-binary and inclusive, rendering everything and everyone meaningful.[78] This notion is orchestrated continually in the writings of the mystics, such as John of the Cross, who depict God, in effect, as the energy of the cosmos, "a living flame of love" inhabiting all things and binding them together in harmonious, yet often unrecognized, communion.[79] It is a basic tenet of such seers that direct experience of this divine aura always reveals a God whose care is unconditional, who seeks repentance rather than punishment, and who proclaims, despite countervailing sensory evidence, as Julian of Norwich heard in her revelatory encounters, that "all will be well, and all will be well and every kind of thing will be well."[80]

The notion of faith as compassionate connection to all that exists—so central to much theological speculation and personal religious experience—is elemental to the intentions of this volume but, as the reader knows, not necessarily ascribed to by many in the world of religion. The dualism that habitually carves reality into those inside and outside restricted social formulations is just as present among members of the various denominations as it is in the hermeneutical framework of the medical materialist, the behaviorist, or the political and economic policies of a market-driven ethos. In her research, Marcia Webb cites a study of American Pentecostals asked to select from 32 possible causes leading to mental psychosis. The three most often cited were disobeying God's commands, lack of faith, and demonic possession.[81] Vacek claims that "Christians are prone to deploy culturally shaped and anthropocentric logic." Even though Christian anthropology is predicated upon the fundamental goodness of all created things, she asserts that many "ingest and adopt modern American social norms that indicate that only *some* of creation is good."[82]

While prophecy may, in some instances, succumb to such dualist and dismissive formulations, its biblical roots and, often, its contemporary manifestations, complement, rather than contradict, the inclusivity of faith and transcendent experience as we develop them here. For, despite its vociferous critique of the dominant classes in a world densely populated with the starving and the socially irrelevant, it is, in its origin and intent, a call to conversion. In its religious manifestation, it laments the fate to befall the hard of heart and does not glory in what might be called their ideological captivity to epistemic structures that make a necessary divide between friend and foe, the sane and the insane, the free and the imprisoned, or, for that matter, between the saved and the damned.

Ann and Barry Ulanov attest that religious faith offers competing narratives in relation to primordial experience. They use the terminology of true and false containment to depict these different accounts. The former, they argue, gives the ineffable "a place and a state of being in which *it* finds itself at ease with us and *we* find ourselves at ease with it. In false containment, religion gives primordial experience such a threatening appearance that there is nothing we can do but flee from it."[83]

Continuing with the inclusive reading of faith, unlike depth psychologies that attempt to understand the neuroses or phobias that confront specific individuals, faith seeks, as we will see with Kierkegaard, to embrace life in all its inner and outer manifestations.[84] In the thought of Rohr, no less than for Kierkegaard, an inescapable part of life in its entirety is suffering. All too commonly, personal losses, unforeseen calamities, and physical pain are cursed, repressed, or turned into an explosive rage; one that almost inevitably takes its vengeance on those least capable of resisting its onslaught. This is true in cases of bullying and domestic abuse just as it is in attitudes and policies that victimize the poor, the homeless, and the mentally ill. When, however, pain is embraced in an inclusive system of faith that recognizes all the events of life, however daunting, as grace-filled and potentially healing encounters, it transforms the soul, increasing its capacity for compassion and forgiveness. Alternately, in defensive and blameworthy ideologies (false containment), all pain that has not been so transformed will inevitably be imposed upon someone else.[85]

St. Bonaventure perhaps expresses most poetically not only the notion of faith as we have portrayed it but also the entire underlying essence of the porous worldview that is at once the domain of the mystic, the prophet, and, to a significant degree, the "mad" schizophrenic. The experience of unconditioned being whose touch they frequently claim to have felt and whose message they claim to have heard is "pure and absolute … the origin and the final cause of all." It is "entirely within and entirely without all things and, therefore, is an intelligible sphere whose center is everywhere and whose circumference nowhere."[86]

Sartre's exposition, *sans* the theological emphasis, pays an oblique tribute to Bonaventure: "Consciousness is the revealed-revelation of existents … Nevertheless, the primary characteristic of the being of the existent is never to reveal itself completely to consciousness. An existent cannot be stripped of its being; being is the ever-present foundation of the existent; it is everywhere and nowhere."[87]

Can any of this be proved? Is there an inherent and irrevocable union of spirit and matter, of the living and the dead, of all with all? Pragmatically speaking, no. That is why we speak of faith or revelation rather than scientifically verifiable fact. As Kierkegaard will suggest in the next chapter, a leap is involved to enter this world—one that makes all the difference in turning the hidden despair in an energetically controlled, nervous ambience of trepidation and exclusion of the ethereal, into an encounter with a hidden wholeness that encompasses the entire universe. One that also communicates relentlessly, through unlikely and usually maligned spokespersons, on behalf of those whose inherent sacredness has been denied.

Conclusion

We have seen in the metaethical exposition just presented that an "ultimacy" that precedes rational calculation is necessary for the construction of any worldview to provide the basic grammar with which its rational and moral contentions are expressed. For instance, there are binary linguistic patterns often found in religious discourse, as Durkheim argued long ago, to separate the sacred and profane, the clean and unclean, the good and the bad, and perhaps, by extension, the lucid from the lunatic.[88] We have devoted a significant amount of attention in this chapter to similar binary patterns in scientific discourse. This was done not to negate the inestimable importance of technical investigation and its effect on common forms of perception, only to stress that it cannot function without starting points that are dogmatic statements of belief (paradigms). In its own dimension, it thus mirrors the "belief" of any dyed in the wool evangelist or, for that matter, prophetic clairvoyant.

The reality of the power of worldviews and their primary basis in a set of reflexive beliefs is revealed in the metaphysical aura that surrounds the authority of science in our culture. Not a few authors have recognized this reality as a new quasi-religious dogmatism, a doctrinaire hegemony of final authority that was once the sole domain of the religious hierarchy. Harvey Brenner writes of a "medical priesthood" that has now replaced the traditional cleric in former theocratically oriented cultures: "We now turn to the physician, the healer of society, as one who is knowledgeable in the ways of science, rather in those of divine intervention, in the hope of dealing with every possible affliction."[89] Branson even suggests that so great is the reach of the medical ideology that it has assumed the same role as former state religions: "[I]t has an officially approved monopoly of the right to define health and illness."[90] Jaspers seems prescient in his warning that psychotherapy, at the time in which he wrote, a new discipline, "has *its own dangers*. Instead of bringing help to people in distress, it may become a kind of religion … a substitute for metaphysics … for faith and assertiveness, or a substitute outlet for unscrupulous drives."[91] Rieff sees the sacred dimension in which science resides as fomenting the emotivism about which MacIntyre speaks. He suggests that its positivist credo features an inherently nihilist (emotive) dogma exhibited without a "note of apprehension" in which, unlike our predecessors, "we can live freely at last, enjoying all of our senses … in a technological Eden."[92]

Despite what appear to be the irreconcilable starting points of the two systems we have briefly surveyed, the prospects for a reconciliation of perspectives are far more advanced than many might suppose. Particle physics and quantum mechanics have, over the last century, amply demonstrated what Whitehead and Rohr call the coherence of everything: the dynamic relation of each with all, from the most minute elemental forms to those most visible in the universe.[93] If, indeed, the quest of science is to understand the relation of things to one another, then, in reference to Einstein and Heisenberg, Bernard Lonergan notes that "it has taken modern science four centuries to make the discovery that the objects of its inquiry need not be imaginable entities moving through imaginable processes in an imaginable space-time."[94] Callahan writes that much of conventional medicine and research has failed to keep abreast with advances in the fields of science, such as those to which we have just alluded, since current medical practice is still based upon a Newtonian model, "while physics itself has become much more complex." A more wholistic understanding of what is empirically strange would reveal that the claims of believers and visionaries will by no means appear outlandish: "The universe appears to be much weirder and more holistically constituted, at least at the micro level, than the assumptions of the Newtonian worldview."[95]

From this perspective, what is termed mental illness, despite the way it is currently diagnosed and "treated" is far more than an individual phenomenon but rather must be viewed often as a broad category of social, ethical, and even cosmic interaction. It is of course far easier psychologically and structurally to allow its "bizarreness" to render it an individual aberration. Yet, as convenient as that might be for the inertia built into social practice and the current canons of common sense, its complexity is begging for richer, unitive insights than those provided solely by the currently honored postulates within the scientific and, by extension, practical domain.[96]

It is also easier to continue "as if" the current dominance of the biological and behaviorist paradigm is impregnable. Jaspers poignantly directs our attention to what he perceives to be the onerous pitfalls of such a stance. He opines how difficult is the task to expose ourselves to the panoply of reality in all its complex and, often, uncharted manifestations, for it requires "constant self-denials, continuous effort, and painful experiences and insights." There is, therefore, a strong urge to withdraw from reality, to find a way "to circumvent it, screen it off, or find some substitute" to surrender to "easy gratification," but such a defensive posture "is always at the price of the loss of one's health or life."[97] In like manner, in his classic text, Thomas Kuhn makes the well-known assertion that "normal science … is predicated on the assumption that the scientific community knows what the world is like. Much of the success of the enterprise derives from the community's willingness to defend that assumption, if necessary, at considerable cost."[98]

Of course, the "cost" to which Kuhn refers is precisely what has driven me to write this book. It is a cost that has helped to underwrite a pervasive and aggressive historical tragedy, played out in handcuffs, prison cells, and, not infrequently, in blood. We have noted that such an uncompromising reliance on the external appears to be less and less scientific, especially given the growing respect for theories in physics regarding the inseparable connection between human consciousness and all the elements of the universe. Still, the old paradigm continues to function largely unimpeded, despite the price it exacts from the vast assembly of human beings who suffer the effects of a worldview deaf to the messages conveyed in the secret language of the heart.

The seeming permanence of the social, legal, and medical structures that countenance this dissection of so many from the social body, as Anthony Giddens has written, may make the rails of the "natural attitude," and the endless social constructions they support, including the current configurations of the penal system, seem so firm and dependable that they are assumed to be "natural." Yet, they are, finally, merely the particular synthesis of function, time, and space. They are reproduced by people like us but are, despite the powerful interests that sustain them, phantasms that can disappear as quickly as people stop supporting them or, perhaps, in our case, as people are able to think those who have, so often, done no demonstrable harm out of the dungeons in which they are forced to abide.[99]

The idea of a harmonizing of frameworks, already alive in so much of the new scientific thought, has been a topic of interest for numerous scholars surveying the psychiatric discipline. Harrington, for one, would like to see the "new psychiatry" overcome its persistent reductionist habits and commit itself to an ongoing dialogue with the scholarly world of the social sciences and the humanities: "The goal of such a dialogue would be … that, even as it retains its focus on biological processes and disease," it would seek "to understand ways that human brain functioning, disordered or not, is sensitive to culture and context."[100] Browning writes that it is impossible for any of the therapeutic disciplines to "completely eliminate [their] implicit metaphors of ultimacy and moral images." What is possible is to be aware of this metaethical reality and name it for what it is "without invoking … the authority of science. It can then submit these moral and conceptual horizons to philosophical testing insofar as they appear necessary to orient psychology to the world of praxis."[101]

So, it is perhaps appropriate as we draw this chapter to a close to make an act of faith, remembering St. Paul (Eph. 1:9–10), that there is a hidden wisdom, as old as the universe, whose express intent and unstoppable cause is to bring all things into one on earth and in the heavens. Perhaps, the exciting and unitive developments in scientific theory will bring that consciousness of universal harmony and the ontological worth of everything and everyone into our common ways of knowing sooner than we can imagine. In the meantime, however, we live in a divided world, and among those on the wrong side of the divide are the social misfits, the odd visionaries, each of whom, in various and, often, idiosyncratic ways, proclaim the sacredness of all on earth and in the heavens and who, just as often, continue to languish in enforced silence and isolation. The deeper issues involved in their widespread rejection and confinement will now be explored.

Why Do We Punish the Mentally Ill?

The previous chapter was meant to provide a metaethical framework within which the determinations of social actors and institutions make both logical and moral sense. Within a materialist, behaviorist, or strictly biological paradigm, the odd mannerisms, the seemingly incoherent babble, or the angry diatribe against the established order point to individuals who have not been properly socialized or who have fallen prey to a supervening mental or emotional obstacle. As we have suggested, not everyone who demonstrates these characteristics is a mouthpiece of archetypal forces or an agent of the divine will that summons the prophet to utter a stern protest on behalf of all left to forage for crumbs in a world with so much rampant excess. Neither is the sting of adamant protest or the looming presence of the schizophrenic, often in the unkempt attire, and, not uncommonly, odiferous state of hygiene of the homeless, a cause for alarm simply for agents of social control or for the medical community. There is no need to reduce either the overt or the inchoate desire to remove from view those most find offensive to a single explanation. The fact, however, is that hundreds of thousands *have* been expunged from day-to-day societal affairs and it will be our task in this chapter to discuss what I believe to be the main reasons why this nefarious exodus has taken place. We do not, of course, speak of an Exodus of liberation, as found in the book of the same name, but a deportation into dungeons of misery and, all too commonly, abuse, with crippling, and, often, lifelong debilitating effects. To that end, the present chapter will locate this ethos of harm within three broad categories: the socioeconomic, the psychological, and the theological/spiritual. Since issues relating to the latter are very much a part of the presentation on both social and psychological determinants, they will be included in the sections addressing those two classifications.

Socioeconomic factors

Neoliberalism

The rise of Social Darwinism in the late nineteenth century, as Richard Hofstadter pointed out some years ago, has been a recurrent theme in the American ethos, although it is hardly unique to the United States.[1] This fusion of biology, ethics, and public policy existed in real and inchoate forms even before the "Reagan revolution" (echoed in the administration of Margaret Thatcher) began the systematic dismantling of the sweeping social welfare reforms of the Kennedy and, especially, Johnson administrations. Neoliberalism is the current face of the phenomenon; one that has seeped into and transformed the civic, economic, and criminal justice sectors of the domestic order in the US and abroad. As James Crossley defines it: "Neoliberalism advocates individual property rights and free trade, promotes the private sector over the public sector, supports deregulation of the market, challenges traditional manifestations of state power, [and] urges virtually every aspect of human existence to be brought to the market." The stated logic is that such laissez-faire tenets are not simply engineered to lower virtually all bars to pecuniary gain for corporate and financial institutions, publicists and exemplars also claim that the framework guarantees the maximization of freedom, the common good, and the curtailment of poverty.[2]

The results of this virtual *carte blanche* to profit seekers have manifestly lived up to their aim of rewarding entrepreneurs and their investors with gargantuan monetary rewards. However, the other side of the neoliberal dreamscape has by no means provided relief for the "huddled masses." Rather than a dream, a nightmare of crushing poverty has been revealed with the uprooting of untold millions, driven from their homes by penury, political malfeasance, and social immobility into the vast, unstable market of low wage jobs with little or none of the protections afforded to the evaporating pool of organized labor.[3] What has been unveiled, in short, is an economy of extraction wherein "wealth is extracted from vulnerable people and transferred to powerful people."[4] Or, as McCarraher writes: "These assaults on the livelihood and dignity of workers have been justified as painful but necessary steps on the interminable road of Progress, guided by infallible market forces to which we owe homage and genuflection."[5]

To further complement this tragedy, the largesse offered to corporate magnates and bankers has not enhanced freedom and the common welfare but unleashed an unprecedented expansion of coercive state power directed against any at the deep end of the "risk pool" who waver from or rebel against the constricted economic and social options available to them.[6] All avenues of escape from endless accumulation for some and "wage servitude" for most "must be closed, or, better yet, rendered inconceivable; any map of the world that includes utopia must be burned before it can be glanced at."[7]

Weber uses the dyad of "propertied classes" and market-determined "income classes" to accentuate, alternately, the broad and slender paths of opportunity available to the two cohorts. Each path is strictly stratified with one's level of "prestige" marking the relevant point of entry. This "status factor" is represented on the upper road by "economic monopolies" and those accorded "preferential social opportunities."[8] In this environment, the very idea of mutual regard, so embedded in theological ethics, succumbs to a world of endless calculation and accumulation in which "estimation in money prices" and "market struggles" dominate all affairs.[9] The "priestly corporation of grace" and concern for those of low status who occupy the lower road of penury and irrelevance is held in contempt as an "impractical value "lying beyond utilitarian and worldly ends."[10]

All of this implies multifaceted and mutually fruitful collaboration between the economic and political spheres. Only then can the roads to deregulated profit be properly paved as well as those leading to the slum, the projects, the courthouse, and the jail. Decades ago, Karl Polanyi saw the necessity of such a union for the success of "*haute finance*" whose only motive "was gain." In order to achieve this end, it was necessary for economic "players" to ally with governments "whose end was power and conquest."[11] He adds a further group of rudiments central to this alliance: "Nothing must be allowed to inhibit the formation of markets ... [and] only such policies and measures are in order which help to ensure the self-regulation of the market by creating conditions which make the market the only organizing power in the economic sphere."[12] Weber's conclusion is similar yet adds a compelling subsidiary value. He observes that the bureaucratic, rational state conjoins with the economic sector to control affairs, "including the punishment of evil." This heavy-handed curtailment of those peripheral to, or disruptive of the alliance of business and government is accomplished efficiently and impersonally, "without regard" for the persons so targeted.[13]

The neoliberal credo echoes in pitiless detail the Nietzschean "straight jacket" that binds all in fetters of accountability to the economic and political regulators of acceptable conduct. In this, I am reminded of Foucault's "prophetic" warning of the invasive expansion of state surveillance into the "interstices" of individual and social life to detect "the slightest illegality" and enfold its perpetrator in the cloak of delinquency.[14]

What is more, the neoliberal model accepts no blame for the adverse conditions in which so many are forced to dwell and are compelled (almost literally at gunpoint) to accept. This veneer of innocence is accomplished in part by the fact that the national and local news outlets are underwritten by corporate sponsors. Their portrayals of breaking events are shaped by deeply evaluative binaries, not unlike those we discussed regarding the treatment of the mentally ill by the police in the previous chapter. Those frames inevitably contain stark depictions of innocence and guilt, the deserving and the undeserving, and victims and predators. The "system" is never at fault; vindictive emotions are frequently summoned; and all is filtered through "attributions of individual responsibility."[15]

Wacquant contends that the lure of neoliberalism for relevant interest groups is driven by "a politics of resentment toward categories deemed undeserving and unruly."[16] When one looks at the shrinking raw numbers regarding serious criminal offenses, the stupefying numbers in jail and prison, the gutting of the once vibrant social welfare programs, and the massive and growing disparity between those with and without means, it is difficult to quibble with his caustic evaluation. For instance, he points out that in 1980, the two largest agencies in the US serving the needs of the economically vulnerable—those involving food stamps and aid to families with dependent children—were accorded three times the money allocated to the penal sector. Three decades later, the numbers had nearly reversed, with the criminal justice budget exceeding by 200 percent the funds directed to aid the poor.[17] Adorno may be engaging in hyperbole, but his critique of economic and political liberalism and its arsenal of punitive weapons for those outside the realm of "reason" or docile servility suggests something similar to what Wacquant suggests: "Predators get hungry, but pouncing on their prey is difficult ... additional impulses may be needed for the beast to dare it. These impulses and the unpleasantness of hunger fuse into rage at the victim."[18]

We have spoken of a "hyperincarceration" pattern in the United States and elsewhere. The nets of the criminal justice system have been calibrated, in other words, not to entrap randomly but to catch only certain kinds of prey. The data reveals the truth of the claim as the three most relevant factors determining who goes to jail are not the crimes committed but the economic class and race of offenders and the neighborhood wherein they reside.[19] David Garland, in like manner, reflects upon the remaking of the prison "as a reservation, a quarantine zone." Not unlike the logic that propelled the foundational course set by the workhouse in the tragic saga of forcible detention, the penal complex is more and more populated with the "purportedly dangerous" segregated in the name of "public safety." Their complexion and wallet size are the determining characteristics of this mélange "drawn from classes and racial groups that have become politically and economically problematic."[20] We thus reiterate that on the other side of the neoliberal coin of unfettered capitalism are the fettered masses who bear full culpability not only for the conditions in which they live but for any deviation from the stringent imperatives established to keep them in the ghetto or, failing that, behind bars.

This fatal union of social disintegration within the crumbling ghetto, the shading of privation with the color of deviancy, and the shading of deviancy with the failure to conform to the normative constraints created by the powerful is a poignant reminder that the history of incarceration is not linear but circular. Recall the frustration of the business and propertied classes at the hordes of displaced feudal laborers and the concerted efforts to confront homelessness and poverty not with charity or opportunity but with widespread institutionalization.

With such a determined and uncompromising political economy, it should be apparent why so many of the "undeserving and unruly" categorized as insane have sunk into the mire of the penal system. As Pustilnik states: "Because the criminal system reinforces personal and social responsibility, and punishes deviance, social meanings that construct the mentally ill as *culpably* irresponsible could create social value by reinforcing the responsibility norm, at relatively low social cost, against a disfavored group."[21]

Scull makes a similar point. He insists that the principal driving force behind the rise of an aversive response to madness lies in the tenets of neoliberalism with its "ever more thoroughgoing commercialization of existence."[22] Brenner likewise surmises that what is termed criminal behavior by the person judged to be intellectually handicapped is explicitly related to advanced capitalist concerns. Thus "both the mental hospital and the prison might be considered agents of social control" in a fiscally charged environment.[23]

Polanyi wrote passionately about the utopian vision of a market that could fulfill both the dreams of entrepreneurs and investors as well as those of mainstream men and women seeking a recognizable and realizable degree of financial security. He states that such an arrangement "could not exist for any length of time without annihilating the human and natural substance of society" and turning it into a "wilderness."[24]

Colored crazy

We have alluded numerous times to the fact that insanity and incarceration have a color to their composition. In broad terms, Herbert Fingarette summarizes this adversarial portrayal (although, in fairness, he does not make any racial distinctions in his analysis). He writes that there are people who are unaware "of certain broad types of moral condemnation by society," who are "unable even to take these attitudes into account" in the way they conduct themselves. Such persons are thereby "marked out as suffering some psychopathology." They are "out of touch with reality" in the same way that one would be who lacks knowledge of "money, or policeman, and the laws against crimes." Their loss of reason (insanity) dutifully manifests itself in "outlandish behavior."[25] As an addendum to this, one should consider (again) the caveat offered by de Young that the ones who have reputedly lost their reason and are unaware of or are impervious to "certain types of moral condemnation," are by no means a heterogeneous cohort; rather, their stamp of admittance into the psychopathological arena is determined largely by their skin color and their economic standing.[26]

The roots of the racially based inference of madness can be traced minimally into the nineteenth century. The 1840 US census, not unlike the 1890 census about which Khalil Muhammad writes so perceptively, was pivotal in fomenting the, at least subliminal, calculation that black Americans, unlike their white counterparts, were prone to succumb to mental collapse. In de Young's words, that census "provided the fodder for an unrepentantly racialized discourse about madness that would continue for decades, despite the fact that the findings did not hold up to scrutiny." It left "an indelible impression, medicalized with the help of asylum physicians, that for black people freedom was tantamount to madness."[27]

For Muhammad, the 1890 census—occurring a quarter century after African Americans were accorded full constitutional equality—was viewed as a bellwether revealing the degree of successful integration of a liberated people into the current of American life. Ignoring the fact that the data collected belied the racial motivation that authorities so often employed to stifle, control, and punish a largely defenseless population, the sociologists who conducted the study insisted that the statistical determinations were "objective, color blind, and incontrovertible." When the results revealed that Blacks, who represented 12 percent of the population, comprised 30 percent of the prison population, the reaction was concerted and furious: "From this moment on, the notion of blacks as criminals materialized" in the national consciousness. It became a "strategy of communication" whose syntax repeatedly delivered a grammar of inferiority, instability, and inadaptability.[28]

Among the earliest sociological investigations seeking to discover whether there is a connection between socioeconomic factors and the designation of psychiatric disorder was conducted by Faris and Dunham in 1939. The research compared rates of admission to mental facilities from various census tracts in Chicago and revealed that race, class, and location played a significant role in determining who was healthy enough to weather personal stressors and neurotic attachments and who was to be forced into confinement. They report that "rates of admission for severe psychoses and 'functional disorders,' especially schizophrenia, were highest in the inner city and tended to decrease in concentric zones moving out toward the suburbs."[29] Other studies have confirmed the truth of Faris and Dunham's observations.[30]

Prescinding from these statistical revelations, American psychiatrists in the 1940s began to alter radically where they drew the line separating "normal" and "abnormal." The schizophrenic tag, up that point, had been applied to about one-third of those consigned to mental hospitals in New York City. Two decades later that number had risen to more than 50 percent. Whitaker corroborates the earlier work of Farris and Dunham in his conclusion that "American doctors were regularly applying the schizophrenic tag to people who should properly be diagnosed as manic depressive, or simply neurotic."[31] Similarly, both Jonathan Metzl and Anne Parsons chart how racial fears and crime phobia exacerbated the diagnosis of schizophrenia among African Americans and how such diagnostic tactics have "had life-altering consequences as psychiatrists committed large number of African Americans to custodial institutions."[32]

Parsons tells the story of George Elder, a mixed race (Cherokee and Black) vagabond who was picked up by the police for vagrancy in 1942. When authorities brought a charge against him for ignoring his call to enter the war effort, Elder argued not only that he was a pacifist but also that he refused to fight for a nation that systematically declared war on both Native and African Americans. In fact, he expected not to serve the government but that the government pay him reparations for the uncountable horrors committed against his people. He was ordered to be evaluated by a team of psychiatrists who labeled him a paranoid schizophrenic and committed him to a state asylum in Pennsylvania where he remained for 39 years.[33]

To summarize our investigation, in a meta-analysis of research on the topic, Holzer and his coauthors conclude that their "strongest impression" is that the much-studied association between SES (socioeconomic status) and psychiatric disorder is still alive and well.[34]

Depleted social services, police discretion, and the determination of medical experts

We are already aware of the widespread abandonment of facilities designed to address those seen to be psychologically maladjusted. Many of the hundreds of thousands of these discharged castaways have lived or continue to live a hand to mouth existence, frequently accosting passersby for loose change, and enervating virtually any semblance of compassion from the society at large. In many cases, they find their lodging either in open doorways, on subway grates, in the subways themselves, or in shelters for the homeless. We also know that each of these living arrangements is, more often than not, a prelude to the fail-safe arrangement of a cot in the county jail. As one study proposes, it is not cognitive disability itself that is the primary cause of involvement in the criminal justice system. Rather, the carceral response is fueled by "externally-imposed systemic and policy driven changes and deficiencies in the management of mental illness."[35]

This public procedure of rejection, accusation, and censure is more and more present across the Global North and other industrialized nations as the disconnected and destitute huddle in city centers across North America, Europe, and elsewhere. Eoin O'Connell summarizes the practice in Great Britain as a "punitive reaction" emanating from the US that began with the elimination of public spaces for "suspicious" citizens, making it functionally impossible for those living on the street to exist without violating some ordinance. The consequence, as he notes, is that "a disproportionate number of people experiencing homelessness are represented in the criminal justice system."[36] The statistics supporting this "war on the poor," the homeless, and those with mental issues are startling: the National Law Center on Homelessness and Poverty reported that in a survey of 187 cities in America, 33 percent have citywide bans on camping in public, 18 percent have total bans on sleeping in public, and 27 percent prohibit sleeping in specific locations. One-quarter have citywide begging restrictions, 33 percent have citywide loitering bans, 53 percent prohibit sitting or lying down in designated zones, 43 percent prohibit sleeping in cars, and 9 percent have laws prohibiting sharing free food. The number of these laws and the inevitable labelling of deviance that accompanies their violation is increasing.[37]

Given such a repressive snapshot, the police have become central figures in this devolving drama as they are placed in the position of navigating a series of constricted options when they observe or are called to investigate a disturbance or infraction involving the least among us. We have already alluded to the thin level of tolerance, not to mention disgust, among a substantial percentage of the citizenry at the sight of many in the throes of poverty, exposure, sickness, and schizophrenic fantasy who are not only judged to be "bizarre" but also "disruptive, or dangerous."[38] Law enforcement officials, then, have a doubly narrow interpretive window given public bias and the ubiquity of bans on all forms of loitering, begging, and sleeping in public. They may consider civil commitment but, as Levesque contends, "the process of civil commitment is filled with procedural hurdles because many of the available community-based treatment programs will not accept patients who are perceived as dangerous." Given those limited options, the decision most frequently elected is to charge the individual with a crime since it is a "less cumbersome and more reliable way of removing the person from the community."[39] Another study corroborates Levesque's appraisal:

> With the mental health disposition less available, but still faced with a need to manage situations involving undesirable behaviors, agents of social control—police and judges—would a impose criminal, rather than psychiatric definition on an individual's deviant behavior. The individual would then be arrested, often on a trivial charge … and in some cases be detained in jail.[40]

The fact that law enforcement personnel are ill-equipped to deal with mental health issues generally and, specifically, to weigh the cognitive state of the large and growing body of partial citizens, has posed no barrier as they are the de facto authority on a given person's state of psychological well-being. In New York City, for instance, in 2015 police responded to more than 400 mental health calls per day.[41] Furthermore, one former police officer, now a professor, states that the first rule in the law enforcement ethos is "do whatever you need to do to go home at the end of your shift." As we saw with the inordinate number of fatalities of mentally disturbed persons at the hands of police in the last chapter, and in the horrific events of violence by law enforcement against poor blacks in cases such as the murder of George Floyd in 2020, the professor in question affirms that training academies tend to over-emphasize worst-case scenarios in schooling potential officers. This culminates in a cultural bias among the police that they are chronically endangered. They then respond by doing all they can to minimize what they determine to be situations in which their well-being is threatened.

What we are witnessing, once again, is the tendency to criminalize poverty and mental illness, with police on the front lines of this assault. The pervasive ideology of deviance feeds this carceral appetite especially since the mentally ill are not appreciated as casualties of a neoliberal reduction in public health services but as a threat to public safety and comfort.[42]

As was his forte, Erving Goffman commented on the symbolic interaction between the socially marginal and their affluent accusers. He notes that "offenses against some arrangement in face-to-face living" lead a complainant to initiate "action against the offender." Of note, however, "is that for every offense that leads to an effective complaint, there are many psychiatrically similar ones that never do."[43] Veysey and her colleagues have a similar conclusion: "Psychiatric diagnoses are stigmatizing labels phrased to resemble medical diagnoses and applied to persons whose behavior annoys or offends others."[44] I infer here that the authors just referenced are alluding to the divide between the admissible emotional and neurotic maladies of those whose public profile abstains them from revilement and punitive sanction and those whose behavior summons a visit from security personnel. Goffman calls these "career contingencies," the foremost of which is "socio-economic status."[45]

Patricia Erickson and her coauthors give further substance to such contingencies in pointing to a 1992 study by the National Alliance for the Mentally Ill. The report noted the over-representation of those diagnosed as mentally ill in the nation's criminal justice system and provided documentation that "most of the mentally ill arrested have not committed major crimes but rather misdemeanors and minor felonies." They then add that this trend began in earnest in the 1970s. At that time, "the social construction of mental illness began to change in the direction of indicating a defect of morality or will" on the part of the questionable person as well as the societal willingness to make a criminal matter out of one's "failure to conform one's behavior to the social norm of personal responsibility." This policy "made it appear rational to reinforce the responsibility norm by punishing the mentally ill."[46] Levesque similarly points to the trend to "increase the criminal penalties for 'lifestyle crimes' which are typically nonviolent offenses that do not cause direct harm to others but do create feelings of unease among community members."[47]

Our discussion thus redounds back to the previous section on race and our repeated theme of the powerful interests that determine the social reality of both crime and insanity. Frankham reports that the use of non-fatal force by the police in the apprehension of white suspects has deleterious effects on public perceptions of law enforcement, however, "for African American suspects, mental illness increased support for police use of non-fatal force."[48]

Fingarette bolsters the conservative deduction that in matters pertaining to public safety, the burden of proof falls upon the suspect, not upon those responsible for the apprehension of "trouble-makers." He notes that the often-lengthy period of time between arraignment of a defendant and a judicial finding regarding the presumed offense hampers the ability to find a suitable solution to the infraction. Therefore, "it may be of value to restrain the person at least for some minimum period for the protection of society."[49]

Criminal guilt, as we have made apparent, can, of course, be ascertained in another way: subjecting the suspect to a psychiatric examination. Laing claims that one sent for such an evaluation, if "labeled as patient, and specifically as 'schizophrenic'," is degraded from full existential and legal status as a human agent and imaged as "no longer in possession of his own definition of himself ... More completely, more radically than anywhere else in our society, he is invalidated as a human being."[50]

Scull continues this thought sequence in attesting that the labels assigned by psychiatrists "stick in a way lay ones don't." He repeats a common theme that privileged or affluent "elites" have "increasingly sought to rationalize and legitimatize their control of all sorts of deviant and troublesome elements by consigning them to the ministrations of experts ... [who] form the final and decisive part of the screening process." This reflexive response is disturbingly true when those determinations are "backed by the police power of the state." Thus, whatever may be the level of culpability or innocence of a character whose actions strike an onlooker as bizarre, threatening, or dangerous, the psychiatrist has the warrant and influence to "transform his judgments into social reality."[51]

We will give John Lofland the last word in this section. He illumines the origin in the social sciences of terms such as social pathology, social maladjustment, and the umbrella concept of deviance among licensed experts or educated elites who deftly apply such stigmatic diagnoses to single persons or powerless collectives, supported, as we have seen, by both the public at large and agents of control. These markers "carry a value bias and repressed moral judgments," by persons "who put the building of knowledge above all other human values" and manipulate "science for their own ends."[52]

The conundrum of mystical experience

Recall the words of St. John of the Cross that many of those who suffer the emotional trials associated with the life of faith and the yearning for spiritual enlightenment will have an intuitive understanding of occurrences such as the dark night or hearing voices. On the other hand, such trials, subliminal messages, and their resultant effects are fully opaque to one who is a strict empiricist: "Only those who suffer them will know what this experience is like, but they won't be able to describe it."[53] From Vico's perspective, the mysterious and hidden language that is so often emitted in mystical expression possesses three important virtues: to "heighten and enlarge our powers of imagination"; to "inform us, in brief expression, of the ultimate circumstances by which things are defined"; and to "transport the mind to the most distant things and present them with a captivating appearance."[54]

For spiritual writers such as John of the Cross, whose poetry exemplifies the qualities of which Vico speaks, the path of descent into the depths of the psyche is the prelude to an ascent into an expansive faith and a resolution to many of life's inevitable anxieties. Rieff makes a point of noting that the ritual practice relative to a contemplative spirituality "is always a form of unification with a saving agency." He adds that the achievement of enlightenment is based on "inaction" or, in James' terminology, passivity. Yet this is for the seeker and suppliant a prelude to "a climax of inner stability," for once it has been attained, "there is no place to go further down, so to speak."[55]

Not to be outdone in his probing of the mysterious encounters emblematic of a transformative spiritual encounter, Alan Watts points to one of its effects about which we spoke in the last chapter: coherence. Here, all dualist bifurcations of reality such as the divide between good and evil and life and death "are felt as the poles or undulations of a single, eternal and harmonious energy—exuding a sense of joy and love. The feeling may be purely subjective … but it comes upon us with the same startling independence of wishing and willing as a flash of lightning."[56] For Rodney Stark, such "confirming" experiences "provide a sudden feeling, knowing, or intention that the beliefs one holds are true … a special occasion of certainty induced by the presence of a supernatural being."[57]

The prophets of whom we write are exemplars of these supernatural encounters. There is a similarity between the insights and visions they receive and what today we call extrasensory perception. Bruce Vawter asserts that there are "natural forces which we have not yet precisely defined, which account for clairvoyance or second sight, a thing that has been verified among all sorts of people in every age." He concludes that it is fully logical that God would impart such gifts "in calling up prophets from among his people, making them the vehicle of his revelation."[58]

Virgilio Elizondo intensifies Vawter's observation in his conviction that when the poor, the oppressed, and those relegated to the social margins "become aware of who they are in the Lord and begin their struggle for humanization, then the true liberation of humanity has begun." In this dynamic state, "prophecy is not just being spoken about; it is being lived out in ongoing confrontations by the previously powerless of society who now dare to go to the Jerusalems of today's society: city hall, transnational corporations, boards of education, ecclesiastical offices." These prophetic emissaries are "are now coming out of their tombs of substandard housing, disease-infected neighborhoods, economically enslaving jobs, schools that strengthened illiteracy, and churches that perpetuated segregation."[59]

Yet, as we have shown repeatedly, such prophetic language, including what Szasz terms the "proto language" of the presumably handicapped, has been at best dismissed as a distortion and a grand delusion and, far worse, as indisputable evidence stimulating the widely held intent to banish from view those brandishing its pointed message.[60] Szasz further contends, reminiscent of Robert Cover's concept of jurispathology, that these negative reactions seek to destroy any language save that espoused in the positivist lexicon. Indeed, many supposed mental illnesses "may be like languages, and not at all like diseases of the body … Suppose, for instance, that the problem of hysteria is more akin to the problem of a person speaking a foreign tongue than it is to that of a person having a bodily disease."[61]

Jacques Lacan accuses the pervasive diminution of the unconscious in the psychoanalytic treatment of what he terms "madness," especially in the rampant behaviorist climate of the United States. What is lost here, reminiscent of Foucault, is the "Word" that emanates from the core of the patient which "has given up trying to make itself recognized." Rather, discourse is thwarted and the client, "one might say, is spoken rather than speaking."[62]

Psychological stress may thus be indicative not of cognitive or moral collapse but fidelity to the preternatural Word announcing the purposes of God. As we will see in the next chapter, the Hebrew prophets were "maddened" not by personal moral foibles—theirs or those of others—but due to "their alliance with the heart of a grieving God."[63]

Continuing this participative theme regarding the prophet, Karl Rahner, similar to Jaspers, suggests that what we are discussing here is a kind of knowledge which is hidden in the depths of each person, one that belongs "to the very roots of cognition" and provides the a-priori starting point "for all reflexive knowledge in its function of combining and classifying." This inner, mysterious wisdom, as we have alluded, is only received passively yet is "a matter of transcendental necessity." Recalling Kant, Rahner argues that the burden of proof relating to these metaphysical truths, so real and yet so empirically evanescent, is not upon those who receive them but those who call them into question. That is to say, human beings always experience more of who they truly are "at the non-thematic and non-reflexive levels in the ... fundamental living" of their lives than they know about themselves through simple self-reflection "whether scientifically ... or unscientifically."[64]

The profile of preacher, scholar, and former mental patient, Anton Boisen, is particularly poignant given these reflections. His story reveals the *reductio ad absurdum* that characterizes psychiatric diagnoses of men and women who are far from crazy, but often touched by an interface with what Nietzsche calls "the ground of being." Boisen illumines the stark difference between an organic handicap and the religious crisis associated with phenomena such as the inner cognition about which Rahner speaks. He writes that psychiatrists regularly fail to "recognize with sufficient clearness the sharp contrast between them." He urges medical personnel to ponder that those under analysis have not sunk into the pit of surreal fantasy but have been touched by "mystical experiences in so far as they give the sense of identification with the larger fellowship represented by the idea of God." He then concludes that perhaps we "need to learn ... that all auditory hallucinations ... may represent the operations of the creative mind."[65]

Despite these justifications for revelatory knowing, the medical community and its law enforcement and judicial adjuncts hold all the aces in the deck that governs social worthiness. In the interchange between the "mental case" and the psychiatrist, each party "speaks a different language, whose content and consequences he seeks to impose on his adversary ... like all such struggles, it is decided not by logic but by power."[66] That is to say, no matter how many times the deck is shuffled the questionable patient always loses.

A case in point is the story of Bryan Sanderson, a middle-class firefighter who, after a series of unfortunate events, including a failed marriage, fell into a manic-depressive state. At that point, he began to hear inner voices. He said: "I thought God was talking to me." The first message told him to print hundreds of t-shirts with the logo "Faith Factor" onto which was stitched a biblical verse. The voice then told him to take the shirts to Texas. On the way, he stopped before three large crosses signaling where a church was being constructed. When he saw people praying there, the voice then told him to give them a generous portion of the money he possessed—$500. With virtually all his remaining funds, again pliant before an audible directive, he rented an apartment building in San Antonio to house the homeless. On his way home, he lodged at a budget motel but, mistakenly, allowed the door to close on his belongings. When his key failed to open the door, in a frenzy, he stripped naked and took the elevator. He was arrested for indecent exposure, the first of his criminal charges. The initial response of the authorities was to put him in solitary confinement. From there began a downward spiral. The punishments, at first, embittered him and he began hearing more voices, these more conspiratorial (such as that the CIA was trying to kill him). After a long ordeal, he slowly began to recover, and now runs a church group for people bearing an uncommon psychological profile.[67] The point here is that Sanderson was undoubtedly bipolar, but he was far from criminal. His story has haunting echoes of both the susceptibility to extrasensory phenomena experienced by many and the categorical way in which they are regularly dismissed as being out of their minds; in his case, despite his eccentricity, for a series of intimations all directed toward the care of others.

Weber states that the tension between religion and intellectual knowledge comes to its highest point when a rational, disenchanted mind or cultural mindset "encounters the ethical postulate that the world is a God-ordained, and hence somehow meaningfully and ethically oriented, cosmos." Those with a practical as well as a "mathematically oriented view of the world" then seek to mute any discourse that elevates the worth, let alone the primacy, of inner experience.[68]

When those whose vision of reality, infused with inner urgings and prophetic utterance, run into the materialist reductionism of state officials, they are confronted by "brutal force" which is "concerned with justice only nominally." It is a power that breeds new expressions of violence "against external and internal enemies" fed by "dishonest pre-texts for such deeds" and, "worse, a pharisaically veiled absence of love."[69]

We close this section with the observations of one of the losers in the mental health poker game: Levert Brookshire. Writing from his cell in an Arizona prison, he recalls that he, and many of his penal companions, derive from "sun-society's low income, government-subsidized, predatory environment." Who are they? "The mentally-ill … nowhere else to live. They are steered into the status quo's penal-system. Where they are converted into a state tax revenue, dependent, joined together with the rest of us, who have succumbed to the mounting social economic, and other pressures. Trying to cope with desperation."[70]

Criminology, net widening, and social control

There are many scholars in the criminal justice field who are as dedicated to the men and women imprisoned here and abroad as they are to the canons of rigorous scholarship. Furthermore, the critique of criminological theory in the following pages, particularly some of the current literature in the area of rehabilitation, is not intended to denigrate the desire to aid those harmful to themselves and others by means of vocational, therapeutic, and educational programs so ably designed and supported by countless scholars and professionals working in our jails and prisons.

Still, as John Braithwaite once wrote, criminology creates crime.[71] What he means is that criminological theory often serves the interests of power and creates the categories, and consequent labels, that are then imposed on a population that in some sense fits the description of the given theory, and in another is made to fit within the parameters of the theory by a host of extraneous factors. We have been discussing some of those factors, for instance, in our just concluded section on the variance in perspectives between the psychic visionary and the psychiatrist; the former, often perceived as delusional, if not dangerous to the medical expert, is regularly dispatched to custodial supervision.

I will concentrate my critique in this section on rehabilitation as it still has a noble ring in the nomenclature of organizational perspectives. Many assume it serves to advance the humane alternative to the patently violent assumptions that underlie retributive theory, the pleasure/pain logic of deterrence, and the employment of selective incapacitation. Since the theories just mentioned are manifestly designed to punish/incapacitate lawbreakers, a detailed analysis of their "talking points" will take us too far afield in our aim in this chapter to probe why we punish the mentally ill, as those approaches are already embedded in the punitive dynamics we have discussed since the rise of the system of enforced confinement.[72]

Rehabilitation, or what many criminal justice scholars call desistance, is, in its current makeover, the most deceptive of the principles governing both the theory and exercise of criminal detention. It shares unique ties to the themes we have thus far addressed as it relies in most of its current incarnations on the very therapeutic perspective which has had such a pronounced effect on the incarceration of so many of those designated as socially and psychically difunctional.

The student of penal history knows that rehabilitation provided the mythology for criminal justice beginning with the opening of the Elmira Reformatory in 1876. It continued to inform policy decisions until it ran aground in the early 1970s due to a host of instrumental factors, not the least of which was the social and racial unrest of the 1960s. That formative ideology, summarized by Garland as penal welfare, in which the interests of society were assumed to be congruous with those of the confined, was summarily demoted and largely discarded in favor of a focus on "just deserts" and, later, deterrent and incapacitative strategies.[73]

Proponents of rehabilitation, none more erstwhile than Francis Cullen, never tired of promoting it as the most benevolent and effective vehicle for diminishing criminal activity. It was not he, however, who was to ride the white horse into the arena and capture the attention of criminal theorists and program enthusiasts with a new appreciation for how the practice could significantly diminish the lure of lawlessness. That distinction fell to D.A. Andrews and James Bonta who unveiled the Risk, Need, Responsivity (RNR) model in their 1994 treatise, *The Psychology of Criminal Conduct*, the first of six editions. It is a blend of the radical behaviorism of B.F. Skinner and the counseling techniques of Carl Rogers. In reference to the former, the authors write that the theory

> draws upon radical behaviorism for its most fundamental principles in that the factors responsible for variation in human conduct are found in the immediate situation of action. Specifically, these include rewards and costs and those antecedents to behavior that signal the delivery of either rewarding or costly consequences for particular acts.[74]

Rogers assumed pride of place in providing the psychological ballast to keep the theory from a cynical reproduction of pure pleasure/pain, deterrent calculation. His approach is based upon the concept of ethical egoism: a blend of self-help and utilitarianism which maintains that the morally correct behavior is always to seek to promote for oneself more nonmoral good than evil.[75] It is a consequentialist method wherein the individual determines the content of those evaluative categories. As Browning contends, the ethical egoist, "in order to be consistent, is not just advocating this as a moral position for him or herself ... Rather, the ethical egoist is presenting this as a consistent principle for all people to follow."[76]

What these and other companion authors offer is a startling revision of the traditional "welfare" approach. RNR is based upon the commitment, consistent with Rogers, that "there exists a general personality and social psychology"; one that communicates its "conceptual, empirical, and practical" components "across social arrangements, clinical categories, and various personal and justice contexts."[77] Moreover, again in contradistinction to the welfare model, criminal acts are not invitations or pretexts, in the words of James Whitman, to "level up" the individual in the maw of the ravenous penal behemoth but, in his words, operationalize a prevailing philosophy of "degradation" driven, at least in part, by "by the intoxication that comes in treating people as inferiors."[78] From Andrews and Bonta's perspective, a statutory offense, "no matter which ... definitions are employed," is a species of a "general class of behavior that social psychologists have been calling 'problem behavior' or 'deviant behavior' since the 1970s."[79]

From this angle, any confined person, let alone the voluntary or involuntary prophet, is a "problem" and a "deviant" long before he or she is evaluated and treated according to the rubrics carefully laid out by the authors. Criminal subjects embody in brightly colored array the first principle in the three-pronged RNR approach: risk. They pose a significant threat to themselves and to the communities wherein they reside. Those risks involve "anti-social cognition, anti-social attitudes, a history of anti-social behavior, [and an] anti-social personality pattern."[80]

Garland argues that the overall thrust of most literature in the rehabilitative field raises the determination and control of risk to the highest position, including, or perhaps especially, the new efforts spearheaded in the area of desistance: "The practice of rehabilitation is increasingly inscribed in a framework of risk rather than a framework of welfare. Offenders can only be 'treated' ... to the extent that such treatment is deemed to be capable of protecting the public, reducing risk, and being ... cost-effective."[81]

The second facet of the RNR program centers on need. Those designated as qualified to address the problematic individual identify the specific requirements, the fulfillment or alleviation of which will enable him or her to overcome the objectionable behavior.

Finally, it becomes the task of the therapist to assess these factors and tailor a set of interventions, given the social, cognitive, and psychological profile that has been compiled (including that he or she, as per the stated foundational commitments, is "anti-social" and a "delinquent"), that are geared to assure maximum "responsivity" of the client to the treatment being received.[82]

As stated, the theory has breathed new life into the moribund body of the rehabilitative ideal. Cullen boasts that it is much more than a model; rather he lauds it as the new paradigm for rehabilitative efforts.[83] Devon Polashek states that "today the RNR model remains the only empirically validated guide for criminal justice interventions that aim to help offenders to depart from that system."[84]

Andrews and Bonta do their best to balance themselves on a tightrope neither embracing punishment as an end nor abnegating their Skinnerian commitment to the latter's belief that all behavior is "shaped and maintained by its consequences," that is, by reinforcers: those of a positive kind when individual actions conform to expectations, and negative or "aversive" reinforcers when they do not.[85] So while they, on one hand, avoid falling headlong into a retributive void by insisting that there is little evidence supporting "get tough" interventions as delivering a satisfactory deterrent to crime and maintain that "it seems that punishment creates more problems than it solves," they cannot avoid tripping over the pleasure/pain reinforcement obstacle.[86] They write that to insure responsivity for those failing to demonstrate the proper "prosocial attitudes," "[s]tudies suggest that we have to turn the dial to full in order to stop the targeted behavior completely" by the "*immediate* delivery of *very intensive* levels of punishment" with the certainty of "no escape or reinforced alternatives."[87]

They and their supporters are adamant that emphasizing the "rewards associated with prosocial behavior would make the rewards associated with crime less attractive."[88] We are, however, left to ponder, once again, the assumptions associated with negatively branding countless persons—a significant portion of whom are operating with a far different cosmology than one framed by radical behaviorism with its distrust, if not disdain, for the metaphysical. They do so with the hot iron of a universal ethical egoism in which the architects and enforcers of proper behavior assume that *their* worldview, their perception of nonmoral good and evil, is shared by those under their surveillance.

In his critique of rehabilitative treatment, Anthony Bottoms clearly sees the pitfalls of operationalizing a univocal, power laden model of human development and decision making and imposing it as the standard by which rehabilitation or, better, desistance from proscribed behavior is accomplished. He reveals that instead of elevating the downtrodden and the "cognitively backward" in a system in which their poverty, homelessness, and unorthodox behavior provokes an effort to understand and provide remedial services, new forms of delinquency are uncovered in suspicious subjects. The latter are then summarily targeted as requiring "corrective" and, almost inevitably, forcible intervention. He writes that such efforts typically take "more severe coercive action in cases of 'unsatisfactory' home circumstances or 'dubious' moral background." These reductive diagnoses, however, "are made by middle-class workers who unwittingly but systematically discriminate against the poor and the disadvantaged." Such judgments that so often lead to a stretch in prison are often rendered "on the basis of extremely impressionistic evidence which is usually not revealed to the offender, and which he cannot therefore challenge."[89]

RNR is the most acclaimed of the new rehabilitative theories. Others such as the Good Lives Model and the "virtuous prison" have also garnered much attention. I will forgo commenting upon them as the first, although much less wedded to a thinly cloaked retributivism, still builds upon the same philosophical and psychological foundations as RNR, that is, minimizing risk and ethical egoism; while the second reproduces the behaviorist notion of character amendment within a socially conservative acknowledgment that the incarcerated indulged their criminogenic tendencies and have an obligation to conform to the social and legal consensus regarding proper conduct.[90] Either way, the offender (often the prophet) is labeled, prosecuted, and treated since he or she lies outside the dimensions of egoist logic and, by definition, is unable to be rehabilitated save through "turning up the punishment dial to full."

Gwen Robinson has argued astutely that the rebirth of rehabilitation came only by cutting the umbilical cord to its socially progressive past. Its new persona, as we saw with Andrews and Bonta, is, in the first place, "explicitly utilitarian wherein so-called non-criminogenic tendencies no longer merit attention or resourcing precisely because they are not linked to risk." Current practices "have been 'sold' on the basis that they exist to promote the 'greatest happiness (or, more precisely, safety) for the greatest number,' not (primarily) the individual welfare of the offender."[91] Robinson further contends that the new formulation we have been discussing is "managerial" in that it has survived by mirroring the concentration upon supposed threats to public safety in all operative criminological theories. Thirdly, it is "expressivist" in that "rehabilitative sanctions and interventions have entered a new discursive alliance with punitiveness ... [they] are characterized by a renewed interest in the moral consequences of offending."[92]

In their trenchant ode to the new penology, the characteristics of which Robinson has enumerated, Malcolm Feeley and Jonathan Simon add emphasis to the demotion of social mobility in the rehabilitative construct with the ascendance of a finely tuned mechanism to identify the risky and keep them in various forms of punitive segregation (they refer to the philosophy of contemporary corrections in one memorable line as "waste management"). Ironically, the clearest sign that the system is functioning properly is not the financial and social improvement of those whose future forecast is clouded with structural constraints, but their continued recycling through the doors of the court and the local jail.[93] As Marie Gottschalk writes, we have dissected the population and those cut off from significance have become "partial citizens" and "internal exiles."[94] We thus continue to punish people whose cognitive and political frameworks fall outside the restricted confines of the "sane" and the acceptable; and we have a disturbing reminder that criminology continues to create crime.

Psychological factors, projection, and scapegoating

Projection and scapegoating

We will begin our exposition of the psychological factors that turn the punishment wheel in the direction of and over the bodies of those seen to be in cognitive disarray with a short summary of Rene Girard's well-known thesis regarding scapegoating.

Girard argues that the cause of all violence is mimetic rivalry for mutually desired objects. Thinking of our exposition in the last chapter on the prevalence of emotivism and the insatiable will it unleashes, particularly in a fetishized, commodity driven market (not to mention a litigious culture), internecine conflicts are rife. As the tensions arise between discrete actors, or between rival groups, the combatants seek a third party, a "surrogate victim," who they surmise is the true cause of their acrimony and they proceed to vent all their venom upon that person or group. This is the origin of the scapegoat.[95]

It is essential for the cause and evolution of reactive violence that the scapegoat, though innocent, is believed to be the real cause of the anger and unhappiness that plagues the rivals. Also important for our purposes is the victim cannot be from the privileged classes, as his or her prosecution, or judicial murder, would provoke a concerted rage from the family and loved ones of the injured party. Thus, Girard argues that scapegoats are always from the poorer classes, typically prisoners or those from the lowest social stratum.[96]

In primitive cultures, there were periodic rituals of sacrifice wherein, according to prescribed rites, a scapegoat would be offered to the god or gods to make amends for whatever was believed to be the cause of communal unhappiness and conflict. Her or his death would temporarily relieve the bloodlust infecting the assembly who would then return to their daily activities. At which point the process would begin anew, slowly bringing to a boil mimetic desires and skirmishes until a new sacrificial victim was called upon to assuage their fear, anger, and the unhappiness of their lives.

Lacking these officially authorized cathartic ceremonies in our own context, Girard maintains that there is a greater need for more and more victims, especially given the acquisitive and emotive profile of so many.[97] The "mad," in their personal dismay, their lack of political and economic voice, and, frequently, in their penal garb, fit in exact detail all of the rudiments of the scapegoat procedure: enough like us that they can be a suitable stand-in for our narcissistic rivalries, and yet portrayed as radically other than us. Their demotion, rejection, and banishment then serve the cause of "justice." And, since the persecutors have ignored or repressed their own culpability, this constant ritual of social cleansing can be accomplished without a hint of remorse.

Marcia Webb captures some of Girard's thesis in her contention that the stigmatization of the "insane" is driven by fear of our own psychological well-being.[98] Dubler and Lloyd quote a prison abolitionist, Jason Lydon, who speaks of the "dangerous sacrificial theology" of the criminal justice system which, under the rhetoric of justice, enacts the scapegoat function in imposing "the violence, brutality, and abuse," rampant in the culture, upon the bodies of its "designated victims."[99] For his part, Rieff lays the blame for this dismissal of the marginal at the feet of "psychological man" who flaunts his arrogance inside us "in response to the absent God." Thus, in both the therapeutic and social status quo, the labeling and vilifying of the incompetent and the socially troublesome is not an example "of a wise [person] exhibiting a fool, or that of a healthy [person] examining the sick." Rather, we must begin with the fact that each of us is, to some degree, a fool; each of us is ill; and each of us is mentally and emotionally handicapped. "[U]ntil we can control the shock of this recognition, we shall not be able to assess the character of our age correctly."[100]

With this background material we can now proceed to look at the thought of Kierkegaard in greater detail.

Kierkegaard's proto-psychology

Kierkegaard begins his theological and psychological portrayal of the human condition by asserting that despair is universal, sown into the very marrow of our bones. It is the product of an irreversible and debilitating paradox between infinite possibility and grinding necessity. The human imagination with its power to dream, project, and fantasize is unlimited. Recall Descartes' proof of the existence of God (reminiscent of St. Anselm's): an endless infinity that dwarfs the highest flights of human imagination. For example, let us imagine the most extravagant state of affairs that would fulfill our wildest dreams for ourselves. Descartes maintains that were we to gain all for which we hoped in exact detail, arriving in that place, we could then posit another impossible dreamscape, followed by another, and the process would be inexhaustible.[101] Kierkegaard, who admired Descartes, has something of this in mind vis-à-vis the limitless realm of possibility.

On the other hand, we live within this mortal coil. Remember the four sightings of the Buddha: all who are now young will grow old; all who are now healthy will become ill; all who are now living are going to die; and all that we possess will eventually be lost to chance, ruin, robbery, or to those who divide the spoils after our death. This is the realm of necessity.

Kierkegaard first describes the despair to which we succumb by overindulging our sense of possibility while ignoring or repressing the haunting realm of the inescapable:

> The self is just as possible as it is necessary ... Inasmuch as it is itself, it is the necessary, and inasmuch as it has to become itself, it is a possibility. Now if possibility outruns necessity, the self runs away from itself, so that it has not necessity whereto it is bound to return—then this is the despair of possibility.[102]

Furthermore, the self that is enmeshed in this form of despair is steadfastly resolute in maintaining the illusion of invulnerability to the sands of time and the whispers in the wind of the fleetingness of all things. The soul in this state plunges wildly into the world and "permits itself to be defrauded by the 'others.'" Like Heidegger's "they self" or the Nietzschean portrait of the servile who bow to the whims of those who define normalcy and acceptability, such a person becomes

> engaged in all sorts of worldly affairs by becoming wise about how things go in this world, such a man forgets himself, forgets what his name is (in the divine understanding of it), does not dare to believe in himself, finds it too venturesome a thing to be himself, far easier and safer to be like the others, to become an imitation, a number, a cipher in the crowd.[103]

In Berger and Luckmann's portrayal, the fickleness of fate, chance, and fallibility, the ominous specter of raw necessity, trigger the construction of a symbolic universe that presents itself most clearly in its "fundamental terror-assuaging character." This is accomplished by elevating "the paramount reality of everyday life" and an institutional order that erects a "shield against terror."[104]

Ernest Becker testifies to this notion concerning the worldly and the comfortable who are locked "inside the prison of their character defenses." No less than the prisoners under lock and key, everyday captives who forever eye an Oz of endless good fortune "are comfortable in their limited and protected routines, and the idea of a parole into the wide world of chance, accident, and choice terrifies them." In the "prison of one's character" one can continue to tend to the illusion "that the world is manageable, that there is a reason for one's life, a ready justification for one's action."[105] The anguish for one caught in this narrow dimension is the result of "not willing to be one's own self."[106]

On the other hand, the second expression of despair belongs to the "fatalist." This is the person who has lost a sense of her identity in the world because, in Kierkegaard's words, for her "everything is necessary."[107] The abject conditions of life, or simply the way in which such a person perceives the run of events, leaves her trapped in a gloom over the seeming futility of weathering the inevitable descent into sickness and oblivion. Overwhelmed by too much necessity, she is far more apt than her fellows to succumb to depressive psychosis.[108] Yet, for Kierkegaard, the one mired in this state is indeed suffering from hopelessness; but it is the hopelessness of "willing to be one's own self."[109] Remembering Durkheim and, once again, Berger and Luckmann, such souls are embroiled in a world of *anomie* (ontological and social instability). To abide in this environment is to be deprived of the shield that enfolds the world of possibility and "be exposed alone to the onslaught of nightmare."[110]

For our purposes, there are many whose bitter life conditions, whose anomic rootlessness and insecurity, force them to confront their fragility and mortality and project them into fantasy. Often, in such cases, the fantasy is not the problem to be assessed and made into a justification for exclusion. The problem is the semi-reality in which they are forced to lodge, their partial citizenship, and the vividness of denied opportunity in a culture in which the rewards for the structurally protected are endless, and endlessly pumped into the eyes and ears of the rejected through merchandising and popular culture outlets.

Becker views Kierkegaard, especially in the exposition just presented, as the progenitor of modern psychology. For the former, the most extreme forms of mental derangement "are clumsy attempts to come to grips with the basic problem of life." In Kierkegaard's disturbing but compelling portrayal of the paradox of our existence, he "is painting for us a broad and incredibly rich portrait of types of human failure, ways in which [the person] succumbs to and is beaten by life and the world; beaten because he fails to face up to the existential truth of his situation."[111]

There is, however, a bright ray of hope and solace amidst this psychological and spiritual wilderness. It is offered to all, but more easily attained by the ones burdened by necessity than those on the success and status treadmill. For the sheltered and well-heeled, their inner gloom is thought to arise because they believe they are "in despair over something earthly." Yet, Kierkegaard insists that their despair is "about the eternal." For to attach such "such great value to the earthly … is precisely to despair about the eternal."[112] It is characterized by the inability "to face into anxiety," to turn away "from newness and broader perceptions and experiences; the closed shuts out revelation, obtrudes a veil between the person and his own situation in the world."[113] For the ones in this condition, there is confusion over the meaning of prosperity and adversity. The latter is seen as an impediment to the possible, but Kierkegaard insists that only "adversity leads to the goal" and, more pointedly, when one reaches temporality's goal of prosperity, he or she "is furthest away from reaching the goal."[114]

Thus, he insists that the only life that one might consider "wasted" would be that of one "so deceived … that he never became eternally and decisively conscious of himself as spirit, as self, or … never became aware … of the fact that there is a God, and that he, himself, his self, exists before God, which gain of infinity is never attained except through despair."[115]

The theologian, Wolfhart Pannenberg, acknowledges this notion of Kierkegaard in affirming that the life of pure possibility inevitably runs headlong into the loss of self-coherence, failure, and "infidelity to one's human destiny." This opens the door to a radical and potentially life-giving consequence: the loss of any credibility in the belief in "human self-fulfillment by human powers alone." Those alienated from themselves "cannot generate their own identity." Any such attempt magnifies the loss of one's ontological bearings, leading to "new loss of self." The way to wholeness and enlightenment for which human beings are designed requires a daring participation in the life of the necessary, with the world, and with the broad range of our human associates.[116]

Max Scheler augments this analysis. He states that the experience of human contingency in an unstable world creates an opening through which one can imagine an order transcending the self. At this point two paths emerge: one can recapitulate trust in the solidity of material schemes by yielding to those who offer security and protection (Kierkegaard and Nietzsche's servile self) or one can "pause in wonder … grasp the Absolute and … become part of it."[117]

All of this returns us to the role of faith. There is no escaping the dread that arises inevitably from the human paradox. Yet "peace and rest" are there to be gained. Not, however, until one "is brought to the utmost extremity, so that humanly speaking no possibility exists." It is then that one can come to know, or better, trust that "that for God all things are possible."[118] This "infinite resignation is the last stage prior to faith ... for only in the infinite resignation do I become clear to myself with respect to my eternal validity." Every person who wills it can train him or herself "to make this movement which in its pain reconciles one with existence."[119]

Recall the idea in the last chapter offered by Rohr that faith unveils the curtain of dread and remorse to see life in its fullness. Yet, the glorious vision is obstructed until one can transform pain or depression through serenity, acceptance, and compassion.

Faith cannot be attained without a leap into the darkness of unknowing. Many consider it banal or "coarse and common work," but that for Kierkegaard is a vast misconception. Faith is possessed only by those with the "finest and most remarkable" of natures. It "possesses an elevation," from which "I am able to make from the springboard the great leap whereby I pass into infinity." In our helplessness we are naked and alone for we "cannot perform the miraculous," but indeed he attests we can "be astonished by it."[120] This movement, this submission, this blind trust "must constantly be made by virtue of the absurd," by the lack of any empirical evidence. He adds, however, that in the process one does not lose "the finite," nor the world in all its splendor and miraculous pluriformity, but "gains it every inch."[121]

The eyes of faith, therefore, have a hue similar to those of the schizophrenic prophet or her radical political companion: their transcendent vision is opaque to those unable to face resolutely both the reality and the cause of their inner instability. Kierkegaard appends the title "the knight of faith" to such fortunate but inveterately misconstrued personages. Compared to Vico's tragic hero who is lauded according to universal sentiments, the "knight of faith has only himself alone, and this constitutes the dreadfulness of the situation." He or she is "kept in constant tension," "is always in absolute isolation," and "feels the pain of not being able to make himself ... [understandable] to anybody."[122]

This is Kierkegaard's essential message: we go through all of life's heartache and contradictions in order to arrive at faith, that we might know deep in our souls that our "very creatureliness has some meaning to a Creator." Moreover, despite our "true insignificance, weakness, [and] death," our lives have "meaning in some ultimate sense" because they exist "within an eternal and infinite scheme of things."[123]

The upshot of this exposition for our message in this book is highly significant. If the foregoing is true, then the definitions of sanity and insanity require a startling reappraisal. The person who posits a reality massively out of tune with the conventional rubrics of life, whose candid confrontation with the inescapability of life's endemic uncertainty and fallibility—compounded often by poverty, racism, and a host of social constraints—and who constructs a reality predicated upon uncommon revelations, suddenly appears to be more finely tuned to reality and more psychologically balanced than her "sane" counterpart. This is especially true if those who demean them are deaf to the inner ruminations of inherent contingency, if they are in steadfast denial of the vaporous transience of all the possessions, prizes, and status symbols that a materialist, emotive, culture lauds as proof of a worthwhile existence.

In consort with the history we have presented, particularly in a Social Darwinist age of wholesale dismissal and, indeed, persecution of the "surplus population" generally (remembering Thomas Malthus), and its prophetic emissaries in particular, Becker notes that the distillation of all of the evil people have "wreaked upon themselves and upon their world since the beginnings of time right up until tomorrow" can be summarized in one phrase: "it would be simply in *the toll [our] pretense of sanity takes*," as we attempt to deny our "true condition."[124]

The schizophrenic, according to Sass, commonly claims to have been the recipient of a transcendent encounter and feels "closer to truth and illumination." One woman's diagnosis of "madness" was a result of her seeing reality "suffused with a bright and preternatural light."[125]

It is indeed true that such persons seem "to inhabit an entirely different universe." However, like religious and prophetic seers across the ages, their vison is persecuted precisely because of the way they have integrated the spiritual and the material in a way that separates them from their public, judicial, and medical judges by a "gulf which defies description."[126] From their side of the shore, it is essential that they reject "the standard cultural denials of the real nature of experience." Additionally, feeling intensely the paradox of human existence, and unwilling to construct "the confident defenses that a person normally uses to deny them," the individual so touched regularly "has to contrive extra-ingenious and extra-desperate ways of living in the world that will keep him from being torn apart by experience" of the real.[127] Their frequent incarceration then belies the tag of insanity and calls into vivid question who is truly sane in our culture.

Thomas Merton, in a prophetic essay of his own, continues this inversion of the question of mental health in an analysis of the trial of Nazi war criminal, Adolph Eichmann. Having been examined by a team of psychiatrists, Eichmann was judged fit to stand trial as he was declared to be mentally and emotionally sound. Merton surfaces the disturbing thoughts that occurred to him upon hearing the medical report. He states that we are wont to

equate sanity with a sense of justice, with humaneness, with prudence, with the capacity to love and understand other people. We rely on the sane people of the world to preserve it from barbarism, madness, destruction. And now it begins to dawn on us that it is precisely the *sane* ones who are the most dangerous.

He then queries what relevance does the concept have if it "excludes love, considers it irrelevant, and destroys our capacity to love other human beings, to respond to their needs and their sufferings, to recognize them also as persons, to apprehend their pain as one's own?" In such a world, where spiritual values have little or no meaning, the whole concept of sanity is rendered meaningless.[128]

Conclusion

In this chapter we have outlined a series of causes for the persecution of the odd and irksome traits that have provided the motive to send to jail far too many men and women on the wrong side of the fabricated divide between the clearheaded and the outlandish.

We began with a discussion of trends in neoliberal/Social Darwinist doctrine that have done so much to reconfigure the world economy into the few enjoying the harvest and the hordes gleaning the refuse. That discussion paved the way for our brief foray into the dynamics of race prejudice in America (not to mention elsewhere) and the nearly two-century-long ideological construction that African Americans were susceptible to mental illness to the exact degree they were accorded freedom, human rights, and respect for their ontological worth. We followed that exposition with the very real constraints that mental health providers and law enforcement officials are forced to accept in a neoliberal world of depleted social services and vigorously expanded surveillance and apprehension of any who balk at the lopsided plane of economic and vocational opportunity. We then reprised some of the discussion in our last chapter on the clash of worldviews that enable those skeptical, if not hostile, to mystical and archetypal experience to dismiss it and those who claim to have fallen under its influence. Next, we took a critical look at developments within the criminological discipline that have provided the intellectual, programmatic, and therapeutic muscle to sustain the incarceration of so many. Finally, we delved into the psychological factors that countenance the pariah status of those labeled as troublesome and crazy with our discussion of Girard and Kierkegaard.

If the foregoing has been to some degree convincing, then we see that the entire social, psychological, and psychiatric edifice wherein mental health is identified and its conditions addressed is infected by economic inequality, racial prejudice, dwindling public services, and flippant dismissal of 2,500 years of religious wisdom. This is aided in no small part by a new criminology anxious to label and stigmatize this population under the tattered banner of rehabilitation and, on a broader cultural note, a widespread denial on the part of many of us of our true condition of blind conformity and a denial of the necessary and terminal limits of our existence. From Girard's perspective, we continue to be lodged within the ancient historical trap of seeking innocent victims for our narcissistic rivalries. From Kierkegaard's position, we cannot tolerate the "mentally ill" who are poor, colored, disenfranchised, homeless, and politically uproarious because they remind us in a fearsome and, at least, subliminal way of our alienation from being, from solidarity, and from the deepest and most real part of ourselves.

The prophets continue to be persecuted in staggering numbers due to injustice, due to the insights that their inner life reveals to them on behalf of all who suffer neglect and senseless violence, and due to a vapid ideology of sanity and psychological health. All of which produce a collective blindness that would rather see the innocent locked away than confront honestly the dilemmas and pitfalls inherent in this beautiful but achingly vulnerable life we live.

A Profile of the "Mad" Prophet

We have thus far outlined how those purported to be mentally ill have been treated both historically and in current affairs. During that investigation, we identified the economic, social, philosophical, and theological sea change that turned the tide of opinion from one of awe, fear, or at least reticence before what appeared to be otherworldly forces, to one of, at best, suspicion, and, much more commonly, a desire to ban from public view the bearers of abnormal conduct. The population remanded to workhouses or asylums in former times, and to jails and prisons now, are inevitably those incidental or perceived as a threat to production, commerce, and bourgeois propriety. Their racial and economic features shape the determinative diagnostic categories that separate their troubling mannerisms from, as we saw in the last chapter, the anxiety and neurotic pitfalls of the materially comfortable in a world of endless possibility.

It is now our task to probe more deeply the contours of the prophetic personality in its unconventional and disturbing guise. We will highlight some of the distinguishing characteristics of these chosen emissaries, linking them, as we have done throughout this study, with the grammar used to categorize those thought to be intellectually handicapped. This will set the stage for a presentation on common sense and insight. The latter is the *sine qua non* of prophecy in each of its historical manifestations since it always exists in a fractious relationship with what is commonly held to be true.

The personality of the prophets
They announce a message no one wants to hear

The prophets who fill the cellblocks and tiers, the disciplinary and "special housing units" of detention centres in America, Great Britain, and beyond, are there, primarily, because they, like the notable "literary" prophets of the Hebrew Scriptures, convey a message that the majority of people simply are loathe to hear.[1] Theirs is, by definition, a "language of newness" and, from

Walter Brueggemann's perspective, it is the intent "of every totalitarian effort" to aggressively banish that language.[2] Recall St. Stephen's words to those intent on his death: "You stiff-necked people … you are forever opposing the Holy Spirit, just as your ancestors used to do. Which of the prophets did [they] not persecute?" (Acts 7:51–52). Jesus, speaking to the Pharisees, states: "Woe to you! For you build the tombs of the prophets whom your ancestors killed. So you are witnesses and approve of the deeds of your ancestors; for they killed them, and you build their tombs" (Lk. 11:47–48). Weber adds his voice to the diachronic chorus in his insistence that it should be "taken for granted" that prophecy in its historic manifestation exists "not only in acute but in a state of permanent tension with the world and its orders."[3] Weber further asserts that one cannot read the Scriptures without seeing at once "the hard, bitter and passionately stern temperaments in most of these personalities … without concern for the situation of the moment. They viewed the world as doomed at the height of seeming happiness."[4] Think of Isaiah's commission (Is. 6:10) to "harden the people's hearts" or Jeremiah's (Jer. 1:10) "to tear down, to destroy and overthrow." They preach that only through tribulation for sins against the Covenant can the ground be cleared "to build and plant" (Jer. 1:10) a new, divinely inspired civil order.[5]

Theodore Long continues in his characterization of this ferocious political acumen. For, in contrast to those who set and enforce standards of social conduct, "prophets stand outside existing structures making claims on behalf of transcendent powers." In their outcries, they question the constraints imposed by authoritarian demagogues and seek to stimulate action "to transform or undermine existing regimes."[6] In the words of David Reid, they challenge the social and economic myths "which undergird society's accepted structure [of] the haves and have-nots."[7] In backing "Israel up against the wall," they brush aside any "cheap grace" that would allow the people to bandage their deep wounds by playing games "with lamentation and repentance."[8]

The prophet Amos (7:10) knew well the fury of those bent on silencing an unwanted message, among them, Amaziah, the priest of Bethel. The latter complained to King Jeroboam that "Amos is raising a conspiracy against you in the very heart of Israel. The land cannot bear all his words."

The fierce resistance that Amos experienced would be well understood by Mumia Abu-Jamal, a contemporary prophet with an "acute" and "permanent" bearing of opposition to the treatment of black Americans. Like so many before him, he has fallen prey to the forces who arrest and detain those with a message threatening to the status quo by creating and sustaining a perception of menace, a-sociability, and criminality. As head of the Ministry of Information for the Black Panther Party, he contributed frequently to the party's journal. The reader can investigate the contested issues regarding his conviction for the death of a police officer for which he was sentenced to die in 1981. While imprisoned, he has continued to circulate his writings while the questionable judicial dynamics surrounding his case have galvanized a large audience both in America and abroad. In fact, in 1994, National Public Radio did a series of interviews with him but their airing on the nightly news summary, "All Things Considered," was abruptly cancelled. Abu-Jamal then transcribed the commentaries; and they were published a year later in a book entitled, *Live from Death Row*. His literary efforts, however, were not a cause for celebration of "correctional education" on the part of his captors. Rather, after the book's release, he was abruptly transferred to Pennsylvania's supermax prison, SCI Greene, where he resides to this day. In his words: "Clearly, what the government wants is not just death, but silence. A 'correct' inmate is a silent one."[9]

As a general rule, taking into account our portrait of the prophet, it should be assumed that if we who view or hear them are not embarrassed, ashamed, or, perhaps incensed to the point of seeking the muting of their voice, we are probably not listening to what they have to say.[10] Or, put another way, if the message being transmitted is *not* discomforting and, to some degree, troubling, it is not a prophetic message. And it gets even more complicated with the implied diatribe against lives packed with progressive opportunity made by the weary specter of the homeless who lie on the sidewalk or trouble us for change. Richard Rohr tells the story of walking past a line of hungry street people waiting for a meal in a run-down section of Albuquerque, New Mexico. Someone had scrawled on a cracked and weathered wall: "I watch how foolishly man guards his nothing—thereby keeping us out. Truly, God is hated here."[11] Rohr correctly suggests that the pariah-like isolation of the homeless conceals not only a deep pain but also a piercing social analysis.

George Shulman renders the prophetic mission as one predicated upon the accusation that the "freedom of some" is premised "on the subordination of others." Whether shouted from the housetops in revolutionary rhetoric or muttered in the "proto language" of groans, sighs, and disjointed speech, the prophet is always making unequivocal judgments of base neglect and hard-heartedness on the part of those who, in one way or another, seek to deny or deflect it. In Shulman's depiction, these envoys from on high are infringing on our self-satisfied sensibilities in proclaiming that the problem is not to be remedied by study groups, docudramas, or even feeling guilty, but by dismantling the systemic and psychological edifice that is defective in its consideration of "what (and who) we count as real."[12]

In their "acts of witness and narration," these clarion callers are saying directly, or at least implying, that we, the "sane," are the ones who cannot face life in its naked vulnerability. Despite the confident—shall I say arrogant—claims of medical professionals, criminal court judges, prosecutors, passersby offended by riffraff, and "lords" of industry and civic clout, that this wearisome cohort is delusional, prophets announce, recalling Kierkegaard, that mainstream society itself lives in abject delusion. They raise their harangue against an audience that Freud and Jung might well consider "invested in denial." In their protestations, they are not only empowered by the source of timeless wisdom to render visible perennial truths "forgotten or disavowed," but also the systemic malfeasance of a culture of contradiction that hides attitudes and principles that have been embraced and implemented "in viciously exclusionary ways." For them, even if only transmitted in arcane symbolic acts, those of us in the mainstream are called to individual and collective metanoia for, indeed, it is their implication that we, not they, are the actual prisoners.[13]

Let us look further at contemporary prophetic exemplars whose message is too strong for the bearers of power to hear.

The reader may be familiar with the case of Assata Shakur. While serving actively in the Black Liberation Army and the Republic of New Africa, she was accused six times between 1971 and 1973 for crimes ranging from Kidnapping to Armed Robbery, Attempted Murder, and Murder. On each of the six occasions, she was found not guilty through dismissals, mistrials, acquittals, and a hung jury. She was then convicted of murdering a state trooper in a highway shootout in 1973. Sentenced to life imprisonment in 1977, she escaped from the penitentiary and is now living in exile in Cuba.[14] Her case is indicative of widespread, and often violent, government intrusion into the lives of black political activists. In her words: "Black life expectancy is much lower than white and they do their best to kill us before we are born." Her oft repeated rallying cry is: "It is our duty to fight for our freedom. It is our duty to win. We must love one another and support each other. We have nothing to lose but our chains."[15]

Angela Davis is another black, prophetic activist who was, first, fired from her professorship at the University of California Los Angeles due to her uncompromising critique of the racism that infects American culture. She was subsequently imprisoned falsely (all charges were eventually dropped) due to her radical, public orchestrations of the inhumane treatment black Americans regularly endure.[16] When sent to a jail in New York, as noted in the last chapter, she was initially housed in a unit for the mentally ill. Her protests for this placement, however, were only partially successful: she was transferred from the mental health unit and placed in solitary confinement under maximum security provisions. Perhaps these words from her autobiography capture the essence of why her message was such that it was decided that she must be effectively "buried" to prevent communication with her fellow detainees: "There was a possibility that, having read [her work], more people would understand why so many of us have no alternative but to offer our lives—our bodies, our knowledge, our will—to the cause of our oppressed people."[17]

In her study of the autobiographies of Shakur, Davis, and Elaine Brown, Margo Perkins captures the essence of prophecy in her summary of some of the common commitments she finds in these three activists. Despite the painful hardships they endured for their fervent beliefs, it was the struggle for liberation that always received primary emphasis in their narratives—their personal travails were simply one expression of the common longing for release from subjection—and each felt called to be "a voice for the voiceless" and "to expose oppressive conditions and the repressive tactics of the state."[18]

Kaveny locates all prophetic denunciation within the format of a legal indictment: a most ironic descriptor due to the fact that they, not the powerful "with their hands over their ears" (Acts 7:57), bear the burden of arrest, conviction, and confinement. Prophetic confidence in the rightness, even holiness, of its witness is lodged within the authority of the "law," perhaps statutory, perhaps natural, perhaps divine, but, in all cases, a condemnation of policies incompatible with the common welfare. In their extraordinary revelations, the veracity of the injustices to which they point are, to them, "*beyond* question."[19]

Lonergan would depict the contemporary socioeconomic and political order that will not hear nor countenance what the prophet announces as a "cosmopolis." Reminiscent of Weber's impregnable bureaucratic labyrinth, it is neither a class nor a state, but stands above all countervailing claims and personages and "cuts them down to size." It commands that its dicta be followed to the letter, none more than its overarching claim that it "commands [the individual's] first allegiance." It is a power source "that is too universal to be bribed, too impalpable to be forced, too effective to be ignored." It is the quintessential example of the totalitarian effort to destroy "the language of newness."

When O'Brien tortures Winston in *1984* because the latter denied that 2X2=3 or 5, or whatever the party commands, Winston, defeated and exasperated, finally concedes that whatever the party says is correct. To which O'Brien replies: "Sometimes it is not easy to become sane."[20]

I think it is fair to conclude that the price of being rendered sane is one that far too many of us have paid to avoid, like Winston, the painful consequence of "speaking truth to power." Brueggemann, for instance, chides the religious denominations in America for an enculturation to "the American ethos of consumerism" that has suppressed the initiative to believe in or act from a prophetic perspective. Their "consciousness has been claimed by false fields of perception and idolatrous systems of language and rhetoric" that lack either "energizing memories" or "radical hopes" since such a bold revival of the same would be not only a curiosity but, more to the point, a threat in the common culture.[21]

In like manner, James Crossley provides a biting commentary on the feckless accommodation of liberal Christians to a rights-oriented mandate, as opposed to one incensed and outraged at the grinding of dispensable humans by the millstone of the economic and political machine. They are devotees of the liberal biblical interpretive tradition that arose with the rise of the Enlightenment, one focused on "freedom of conscience," "rights, law and consensus." In this scandalous hermeneutic, the preaching of Jesus is scanned to produce proof texts to assure the comfortable and affluent that the Bible and Jesus represent true democratic ideals while, at the same time, vilifying the prophetic actions leveled against that summation as "undemocratic, tyrannical, and terroristic."[22]

In this opening section, we have contended that the integrative and disquieting message of the prophets is an outrage to the grammar and organizational colossus of profit, power, and an ideologically indifferent, if not hostile, populace, which includes many religious adherents. The voices from the margins are reduced to the status of rebels whose freedom of speech and assembly must be consistently repressed.

This now brings us to the second of our traits that define the identity of this troubled and troubling assembly: they are overwhelmed, seduced, and charged by a transcendent source to bear the painful cross of giving voice to the pain of the voiceless.

They are chosen and compelled to speak on behalf of the oppressed

Weber writes: "The prophet could never arrive at a permanent peace with God … The prophet could only discharge his [or her] internal pressure."[23] This suggests Von Rad's conclusion that all prophets are visionaries who, in theological terms, receive an overpowering command "personally addressed" to them by God.[24] For David Reid, "the Word" became their "lot in life and the opposition to God's Word made a passion narrative of the prophet's human existence."[25] The words of Jeremiah (20:9) best exemplify the notion of dis-ease and fruitless protest provoked by that illuminating encounter and its intimate, compelling, and over-powering summons: "But if I say, 'I will not mention his word or speak anymore in his name,' his word is in my heart like a fire, a fire shut up in my bones. I am weary of holding it in; indeed, I cannot."

The prophets we have met, and will continue to meet in our exposition, are, from this perspective, doubly burdened: not only punished by their audience because their message is so threatening and offensive, but also helpless to resist its presentation to inhospitable people with "a hard forehead and a stubborn heart."[26] This onerous state of affairs is different, though not antagonistic to, the highs and lows experienced by the mystic. While the latter hungers for and deliberately seeks union with the divine, Heschel contends that the revelation received by the prophets is often one they would, under normal circumstances, refuse to embrace. It saddles them against their will; it is "not a favor … but a burden."[27]

Indeed, none of the classical prophets claimed to be a mystic or "in possession of holiness." Each was no more than a "a means of communication," simply a "tool" for the communication of divine imperatives for social and religious reform.[28] Yet, whatever the trauma their inner attunement to the divine may bring, their ear, like that of the mystic, remains fixed upon the mysterious calling welling up from within. They are "struck by the glory and presence of God, overpowered by the hand of God."[29]

The Hebrew word *nabi* denotes one who can bear the presence of God as well as the psychological and social degradation shown by those to whom God has chosen her to speak. Martin Buber shares that in ancient Israel, the term, as we have noted previously, was dramatically different from that of a temple seer or shamanic diviner. The *nabi* does indeed include the role of seer and diviner, receptive to primal forces, but, above all things, her task is to be a transmitter of vital messages from, as it were, heaven to earth. The future is indeed wide open and the *nabi* is impelled to "set the audience, to whom the words are addressed," before an imminent choice and decision.[30] Karl Rahner would call such a person a "witness" who calls upon "the freedom of the hearer" to make "the ultimate decision" regarding one far greater than him or herself.[31]

One might think here of the double-edged sword wielded by the prophet in terms of the sentinel metaphor in Ezekiel (33:7–8). He has been appointed "as a sentinel for the house of Israel." When he hears a word from the mouth of YHWH, he must sound a warning; otherwise, he will suffer the same fate as those whose ways have prompted the godly intervention: "When I say to the wicked, 'wicked, you must die,' and you do not speak up to warn the wicked about their ways, they shall die in their sins, but I will hold you responsible for their blood."[32] Joseph Blenkinsopp uses the metaphor of an antenna to portray someone like Ezekiel who serves as "an early warning system" with a message that has life and death consequences for all involved, including him or herself.[33] In this vice of both internal and external pressure, how could one welcome such weight and liability with joy or equanimity?

Our presentation to this juncture, with its long line of accursed ambassadors, loudly affirms the insights just recorded. Their calling is "distasteful" to them "and repugnant to others."[34] Yet, despite the strains and seeming hopelessness of the mission with which they have been charged, they, in effect, magnify in their words and gestures the claim of Habakkuk (12:4) concerning YHWH: "Your eyes are too pure to bear evil; you are unable to look at oppression."

Consistent with the harshness of their life circumstances and that of those for whom they speak, prophets of the street always convey their message in " 'this-worldly' categories," bypassing pleasantries and erudition in favor of profane speech. Von Rad observes that the very nature of their subject matter demands "nothing short of a bold method of expression ... simply because the prophet's message thrust out at every side beyond each and all of Israel's sacral institutions."[35] The very urgency of the rapidly accumulating symptoms of social and human decay, then as now, demands the use of readily available colloquialisms.[36] The focus is *always* on the here and now, of an ominous reality whose portents are fully on display. As with "all good preaching," it is eminently pragmatic.[37] They make use of secular images "with exactly the same freedom as with religious ones, as if there were no difference at all between them."[38]

A street prophet of our own day, Assata Shakur, displays this vernacular approach. She employs powerful idiomatic verbiage to carry her critique that must have had its equivalent in the millennium before Christ: "If you are deaf, dumb, and blind to what is happening in the world, you're under no obligation to do anything. But if you know [or, perhaps, sense] what's happening and don't do anything but sit on your ass, then you're nothing but a punk."[39]

The communicative tropes that Shakur, like her great predecessors such as Amos, Jeremiah, and Ezekiel, employ place her in judgment against her own kith and kin.[40] This oppositional and adamant independence hearkens back to the distinction from prophets attached to the throne, for there was "no place in the cult for the idea that Yahweh would enter into judgment with his own people."[41]

The daunting yet essential revelatory role of prophecy traces back to the very beginning of Israel, whose very existence and endurance of formidable trials in Egypt and the sojourn in the desert were predicated upon acts of supervening mercy and grace. If Israel abandoned its fealty to YHWH, it would lose the support essential for its very survival. The prophet was (and is) the lifeline, the umbilical cord, fashioned to connect a forgetful and idolatrous people to the source of its very life. In this climate, fraught with momentous moral decisions, "the saving God" must now exercise the role of "the judging God." There could be no further salutary intervention from the Creator without attention to the stern and sobering judgments uttered by the prophets on behalf of the widow, the orphan, the alien, and the poor.[42]

Martin Luther King refers to the ancient prophets in proclaiming that he engaged in agitation and nonviolent protests, and suffered scorn, threat, and incarceration (in this case in Birmingham, Alabama), for no other reason than "injustice is here." He states that "just as the eighth century prophets left their little villages and carried their 'thus sayeth the Lord' far beyond the boundaries of their hometowns ... I too am compelled to carry the gospel of freedom beyond my particular hometown."[43]

In his summation of Buber's account of the "theopolitics" of the prophet Isaiah, Walzer follows King's own estimation of the gravity of the hour and reprises the regular prophetic refrain that it is fanciful to think that entering into negotiation or alliance "with the powers" can bring an end to entrenched systemic bias. Moreover, he maintains that such compromises serve to renounce "the power of powers" and, in consequence, serve to sever the ties that lead to divine sustenance. As such, Walzer takes issue with Buber's conclusion that Isaiah is seeking a new "political understanding." Rather, he contends that the prophet is calling for "a radical withdrawal from politics" as a strictly "geopolitical" solution as opposed to full trust in the covenant established with YHWH.[44]

These judgments of impending social cataclysm for the idolatrous are still made against what the prophets insist is a life-affirming and fully realizable vision. They announce the coming judgment of national disgrace and ruin not in smug self-righteousness but in an appeal to the governing authority to forestall its arrival.[45] The people are in a "place of supreme crisis, indeed almost a place of death," and the holes in the communal fabric cannot be mended "by the saving force of the old appointments," only by turning in faith toward the divine handiwork.[46]

Yet, their assurance in the promised deliverance from human malevolence and civic catastrophe does not stem "from any misplaced confidence in human determination and calculation."[47] Indeed, no prophet would deny the myopia, violence, and prideful tenacity of the temporal order. However, this concession, recalling Isaiah, is made only for the purpose of inferring the "radically diabolic character" of that order.[48] What they did believe in was the reality and assurance of a divine reign where the wolf would lie with the lamb (Isa. 11:6), where captives would be set free (Isa. 61:1), and where weapons of war would be transformed into tools to feed the hungry (Isa. 2:2–4). These were realizable ends, given the proper focus on the One "from whom all blessings flow." Within their clouds of social critique, a ray of light consistently shines, insisting that true distributive and social justice are achievable, not because it is possible to overcome the sins of greed, racism, and murderous conduct but due to the reality of "an omnipotent God who could prevail over human weakness and malice."[49]

Given the stakes at hand and despite the burden of uttering it, the message is as uncompromising as the purity of the One from whom it was received. For the emissary is but the reed through which the benevolent force that formed and guides the universe imparts the melody of relentless dedication to, and care for, the downtrodden and forgotten.

Heschel corroborates this instrumental role. He asserts that all true prophets are "bowed and stunned" at the rapaciousness of human greed for they are but "the voice that God has lent to the silent agony, a voice to the plundered poor, to the profaned riches of the world." Indeed, "God is raging" in their words.[50] They are unbending in their call for "righteousness" manifested in "care for the oppressed, the hungry, and the homeless."[51] They willingly take their place with all "whose exclusion makes the whole partial."[52]

For Kaveny, the "bitter and harsh" tone of prophetic indictment cannot be reduced merely to "impoliteness or incivility." Rather, their passionate convictions are based first upon the fact that "knowledge of goodness has been communicated to the human soul by God," that those who find themselves "in a state of wickedness" are "deprived of the power of knowing God," and that they, the heralds, "have been given a special insight into the mind of God."[53]

Prophecy, in this role of announcing a vociferous verdict against self-satisfaction, rendered not simply to condemn but to save, is a constant that is no different in our own day as in ancient times. Whether done in the name of God, or in the name of human solidarity, or in spontaneous words and actions of protest, it riles and provokes in order to announce a new and inclusive reality. That it consistently finds an apathetic, if not vindictive, audience who escort or drag its representatives into bastions of pain, and, most importantly, silence, does nothing to diminish the sacredness of the task.

Writing of the "mass imprisonment" of dissenters in Stalinist Russia, including his own, Solzhenitsyn's colorful words have lost none of their evocative power nor their appalling relevance to the fate of contemporary prophets:

> Through the sewer pipes the flow pulsed. Sometimes the pressure was higher than had been projected, sometimes lower. But the prison sewers were never empty. The blood, the sweat, and the urine into which we were pulped pulsed through them continuously. The history of this sewage system is the history of an endless swallow and flow.[54]

After an anguishing account of the suffering, torture, and utter helplessness of people whose only crime was the outrage their suspected anarchic and "insane" actions provoked from the power of the state, Solzhenitsyn discloses his loss of a satisfactory answer to such degradation: "How can you stand your ground when you are weak and sensitive to pain …? What do you need to make you stronger than the interrogator and the whole trap?" He then states, presumably to other prophetic figures whose imprisonment cannot be equated in any meaningful way with destructive or malevolent conduct, that from the moment the cell door closes, you must say to yourself:

> My life is over, a little early to be sure, but there's nothing to be done about it. I shall never return to freedom. I am condemned to die—now or a little later. But later on, in truth, it will be even harder, and so the sooner the better.[55]

Are we, thus, to conclude that the costs of witness to the truth overpower whatever meaning the prophet may derive from resisting the current of the mainstream that carries with it violence and the violent subjugation of dissent? That is an answer only the prophet can answer. But there is no doubt that her ear is acclimated to impulses far more compelling than the routine cadences of commercial and conventional interchange. She hears and brings to the world's ear "the silent sigh."[56]

The prophet is a creature of solitude

While, as Heschel claims, the prophet ordinarily is not a mystic in the classic sense, namely, one who, thinking of Camus' character, Tarrou, in *The Plague*, "has the least lapses of attention" in the longing to touch and be touched by the hand of God, he or she, like the mystic, moves to rhythms few have learned to recognize.[57] Thus, as Thomas Merton insists, both are "outlaws," seeking resolutely to anchor themselves apart from the those sucked into the vortex of consumption, socioeconomic status, and personal and state violence.[58]

Speaking of his time spent with Indonesian shamans who have the uncanny power to transmit the messages of the natural world to their villages and vice versa, David Abram observes that they "rarely dwell at the heart of their village." Rather, "their dwellings are commonly at the spatial periphery." This is due to the fact that their specialized intelligence "is not encompassed *within* the society." In fact, they are often feared and accused of diabolic incantations yet, the price they pay in loneliness creates the space from which they mediate between "the human community and the larger community of beings upon whom the village depends for its nourishment and sustenance."[59]

Similarly, not all prophets are "knights of faith," as some, or many, do not openly embrace their charge with trust in God or the benevolent powers of the universe. What they share with the former, however, is a profound sense of isolation such as that found in the poor beggar, the inner-city schizophrenic, the bearer of bipolar disorder, and the restless and angry reformer screaming from the housetops for justice. The radical black activist, George Jackson, writes from the prison cell he inhabited from his arrest at 18 until his death at 29: "Why can't I rid myself of the sorrow and emotion that awareness has brought me? I get rid of the self-destructive force of error and ignorance only to be torn and miserable by what I discover."[60]

This profound sense of alienation is compounded by the fact that Merton echoes Kierkegaard in observing that only the ones who openly face vulnerability and death, not out of stoicism, but from a frank appraisal of the affairs of the world around and within them can pierce the outer and inner depths of the field of human experience. Whether in their sensitivity to intuitive, archetypal, or direct revelations or, perhaps, as a result of maltreatment due to their social status or political commitments, these solitary creatures are grasped by the "invulnerable inner reality" that can only come to consciousness when one sees the unreality of the "vulnerable shell" that those insensitive to the inner world try so desperately to maintain.[61] They are then, like the mystic, thrust into the solitude of "the desert" and find there that the "fear of death and the need for self-affirmation are seen to be illusory."[62]

Kierkegaard, once again, was percipient in this regard. He had the same appraisal of the anguish, insight, and social recrimination that characterize the solitary world in which "street prophets" always seem to dwell:

> In the constant sociability of our age people shudder at solitude to such a degree that they know no other use to put it to [except] … as a punishment for criminals. But after all it is a fact that in our age it is a crime to have spirit, so it is natural that such people, the lovers of solitude, are included in the same class with criminals.[63]

The loneliness of the prophet is testified in readings of the ancient texts. This sense of isolation was, for Heschel, typical for one who "alienates the wicked as well as the pious."[64] Buber speaks of Jeremiah as "one among the martyrs of the ancient world." The latter shares his suffering and afflictions with us throughout his revelations just as "he whispers or cries about them to his God."[65] Von Rad references Baruch as an exemplar of the dark night about which we spoke in Chapter 2. For Baruch keenly observed that far more was involved in his role than merely conveying divine displeasure with human recalcitrance. Not only "the prophet's lips" but also the "whole being" becomes absorbed in the service of prophecy: "Consequently, when the prophet's life entered the veil of deep suffering and abandonment by God, this became a unique kind of witness-bearing."[66]

In seeking common elements in eighth-century prophets such as Amos, Hosea, Micah, and Isaiah, von Rad concludes that they "were set apart from their contemporaries and they were very lonely." For they attended to a word and a summons from YHWH "which came to them alone and which could not be transferred to anyone else."[67]

Unlike Moses, whose encounters with the divine illumined his face (Ex. 34:33–35), the later prophets had no such public verification of their encounters with the Holy One and thus lacked any demonstrable evidence of the authority of their oracles. Only the words they spoke, and the verification of those pronouncements in the lives and politics of their contemporaries, could possibly redeem the authenticity of their warnings.[68]

From a contemporary perspective, Russell Schutt writes that this visceral sense of abandonment is associated with feelings of depression and a reduced sense of personal control. It leads to what many would term a "distorted social cognition" and an inability to tolerate the master narrative of the architects and enforcers of the status quo. The result elicits not merely unfavorable "views from and rejection by others," but also "even more social withdrawal and more pessimistic social expectations."[69]

Schutt's conclusions are brought into sharp focus by Jens Soering who, from his cell while serving a double life sentence, relates the isolation and anguish of a transsexual whose given name was Oliver but, belittled and abused after 23 years of confinement, began to beseech penal authorities to be named Olivia. Assuming the new identity and even carrying a purse to the work assignment in the kitchen to which he/she had been assigned, Olivia was forbidden to enter the job site until the purse was disposed of. The affront to her identity led to a heated altercation with authorities and being "frogmarched" into a punishment cell. That night, she mutilated her scrotum with a razor blade in an effort at self-castration and then managed to write in blood on the wall, "I am a woman." The horrifying and evocative symbolism of her protest convinced her captors of serious mental derangement, and she was placed in five-point restraint.

Soering compares the incident to the gospel story of the Gerasene demoniac (Mk 5:1–20) who, similarly, was forcibly bound as a result of his incomprehensible ravings. Yet, he often burst the chains villagers used to immobilize him and cut himself with stones in protest. Jesus travels to the Gentile country of the Gerasenes in the synoptic accounts and not only restores the demoniac to "his right mind" but charges him to proclaim to the surrounding villages "how much the Lord has done … and what mercy he has shown." In his revelatory comments on the loneliness fostered by such presumed insanity, both in the case of the demoniac and Olivia, Soering reminds us of the words written by the apparition of a hand that wrote on the wall of King Belshazzar's palace in the book of Daniel (5:5). The king summons Daniel who reveals their meaning: "You have been weighed in the scales and found wanting" (5:27).[70]

All of this accentuates the point that the experience of separation and rejection suffered by the prophet has not changed; nor has the charge of mental instability; nor has the relevance of the advice that Daniel gives to the king if he wishes to live in accord with the will of God: "O king, may my counsel be acceptable to you: atone for[your sins with righteousness, and your iniquities with mercy to the oppressed" (Dan. 4:27).

Prophets are crazy

Stories of extraordinary perception and accusations of delusion and hysteria have been magnified in the history that we have narrated up to this point. Still, it is important to consult leading scholars to supplement the exposition.

Heschel unequivocally affirms that the prophet is "stigmatized as a madman by his contemporaries."[71] For von Rad, as we have made mention, the oracles uttered are not always in clearly parsed, articulate form. In many cases, they are accompanied by "all kinds of symbolic actions, some of which were extremely odd."[72] The idea they hoped to convey "uses even the most suspect means" to turn the focus of the listener to the distorted reality the usurpers of divine sovereignty have created. This illusory reality to which the apathetic, weak-willed, or consciously malevolent have given their consent must be punctured so the latter can be shocked into seeing the situation that the downtrodden and beleaguered are forced to endure. As we have seen, these mysterious messengers are prone to use "every possible rhetorical device" and are not bashful about employing "extremely radical forms of expression or even caricature."[73]

"Madness" in clinical expositions can be the result of repressed anger; anger that when finally released can take form in wild gestures of defiance and resistance. We have amply established how such outbursts are ridiculed and suppressed but, at the same time, we have stressed that in prophetic communication, such outcries are the necessary antidote for those poisoned by the venom of the "master's discourse." This frenzy takes two forms of expression: the first is revealed in those voices of dissent reacting against the enslavement of the lowly, and the second, in those assumed to be psychotic who exhibit their indignation with the tempestuous gestures born of repressed freedom and equality.

For Foucault, the intolerable histrionics of those condemned to enforced internal exile and confinement reveal that "madness comes from the world of the irrational and bears its stigmata." More exactly, their "crazed" attempts at recognition attest to the fact that there are some who dare to cross "the frontiers of bourgeois order" of their own accord and place themselves and remonstrate "outside the sacred limits of its ethic."[74]

This reduction of insight to madness suggests the work of Victor Turner and the strained interplay between the liminal and the structural. All social systems move inevitably toward fixed roles and obligations with stringent protocols to limit creativity and innovation; the latter are perceived as a threat to the smooth operation of institutions and established norms of order. One may think here, once again, of Nietzsche's emphasis on the anthropological turn from the person immersed in cosmic mystery to one whose words and actions are subject to policing from those in positions of authority. Liminality, however, the literal doorway from structure into anti-structure, is the realm of the possible, the playful, the imaginative, the transformative and is always accompanied by an accent on community (*communitas*). In a liminal state, "we" is the essential trait.[75] Turner says that

> liminal areas of space and time—rituals, carnivals, dramas … —are open to the play of thought, feeling, and will; in them are generated new models, often fantastic, some of which may have sufficient power and

plausibility to replace eventually the force-backed political and jural models that control the centers of a society's ongoing life.[76]

Here we have the explicit domain of the prophetic with all its "abnormal" theatrics and disheveling of the neat social, economic, racial, ethnic, and, for that matter, mental categories that keep everyone in their assigned place. For the ones who occupy liminal space are often there not by choice but by prescribed circumstance. They are literally at the "threshold" of the protected political and monetary interchanges that assure the boundaries of privilege are firmly held in place. Turner states that, in this realm, "symbolic behavior" dominates and further illumines "the detachment of the individual ... from an earlier fixed point in the social structure."[77]

There are, here, lines of connection to the many who then and now claim to be in the throe of subliminal messages, apparitions, sounds, and smells. For instance, there is an international community of voice hearers who bolster one another's integrity and sanity in a raft of mutual acceptance on a sea of "bourgeois order" and abject rejection of their cognitive stability. One such person references Jung and (by inference) Turner, in writing of another

> conscious[ness] that contacts certain humans ... These voices some people hear are guiding us to a new human conscious[ness] or a new way of thought for humanity ... [C]urrently we are a culture that worships power ... all the wars and horrible acts humans have done and are still doing are going to change and the voices are leading us to a better more humane society for all humans.[78]

We have already made the argument that many of the involuntary prophets, the voice hearers and vision recipients, are abruptly labeled as troublesome schizophrenics and, if penniless in a social capital sense, readily dispatched into detention. Unlike the many patients of means and mobility who receive care without shame and metaphorical pollution, with whom "one feels an immediate sense of a shared humanity," the poor schizophrenic "seems to inhabit an entirely different universe; he is someone from whom one feels separated by a 'gulf which defies description'."[79]

We have thus something of a self-fulfilling prophecy: susceptibility to visions and audible revelations renders one isolated socially; this condition then exacerbates the contention of medical professionals that the "outsider" suffers from an abject personality disorder. As Neale and Oltmanns observe, "psychotic episodes," here, perhaps, including the subliminal messages the rejected often receive, are directly related to "an increased rate of stressful events" in their lives.[80] One of the leading American psychiatrists of the first half of the twentieth century, Adolph Meyer, was the first to argue that environmental factors were inherently linked to the development of schizophrenia. He focused on "reaction types" as opposed to reducing the patients' actions to a set of specific diagnostic stereotypes. There was, thus, in his view, a reciprocal relationship between a client's behavioral and cognitive imprint and the inhabited social context.[81] For Laing, one must locate the "cause" of "schizophrenia" not in the diagnosis rendered by a licensed therapist but in "the whole social context in which the psychiatric ceremonial is being conducted."[82]

For its part, the public largely reproduces the hegemonic discourse that justifies the cultural and institutional walls that separate the lucid from the presumed lunatics. As Scull notes, and as we have repeatedly observed, those crazed personages, drawn overwhelmingly from the lower classes and, often recipients of public aid, are "a liability rather than an asset." Employing a geographical metaphor, one finds the "troubled citizen" in a literal and figurative ghetto that distances her and the blemish of her obsessions, neuroses, and susceptibility to voices far from the habitations of respected citizens who often exhibit the same conditions. Consequently, the run of the mill neurotic can rest more secure in her psychotherapeutic treatment without "the socially contaminating effects of overly close association with an impoverished, clinically hopeless clientele."[83]

Prophets are indeed crazy because there is no room for them in an order where all variations of the norm that cause alarm or discomfort to the comfortable are banned and resourced by an arsenal of cultural and institutional weapons of defense aimed to eliminate them and the message they convey.

Prophets are compassionate

There are many angry prophets. In fact, it can be assumed to be a professional requirement. For their very existence, from a theological standpoint, is designated by God to manifest the divine anger at the denigration, neglect, and abuse of the helpless. As we have maintained in this chapter, however, the fountain from which prophetic inspiration arises is one of unconditional love for all. In the Hebrew Bible, there is a constant interplay between obstinate transgression, punishment, and restoration. Heinz Cassirer writes that the passionate denunciations typical of prophetic utterance are punctuated repeatedly not only with the belief that human beings "cannot but become wicked when they turn from God," but also that "in becoming wicked they are inevitably plunged into a state of misery and unhappiness." It is shorthand for the biblical revelation that until God intervenes upon human autonomy and sovereignty, humans create for themselves a state of "spiritual death."[84] Life comes and returns to God and God alone can sustain it.[85] Even more to the point, God *seeks* to sustain it. As a result, that very condition dictates why "letting [people] go their own way is foreign to the prophetic way of thinking."[86]

Of course, one cannot eliminate some degree of healthy self-interest in their calls for reform. After all, as Westermann phrases it so poignantly, they are sitting in the boat whose capsizing they are commissioned to announce.[87] Like the shaman spoken of earlier—marginal to the mainstream but still an essential part of the commonweal—they are mediators between the supernatural and the human world, with the latter immersed in "realities it does not understand or control." Even if unbeknownst to them, prophets are enveloped by a force that longs to "redeem the community they address" and whose fate they are involved in sharing.[88]

Weber notes that the prophetic role in "religions of salvation" is always "fused with a charitable realization of the natural imperfection of all human doings." Of course, given the broad continuum upon which feelings of benevolence can be located, the depth and breadth of empathic connection can vary considerably. Still, Weber insists that the impulse of the prophet "has always lain in the direction of a universalist brotherhood, which goes beyond all barriers of societal associations."[89] In her novel, *Gilead*, Marilynne Robinson uses the book's central figure, Reverend John Ames, to reflect on the legalism of the Scribes with whom Jesus often contended. Unlike the former, the reverend states: "The prophets love the people they chastise."[90]

One sees repeatedly that the prophets, by and large, are not single-minded purveyors of doom. Westermann emphasizes that their messages of judgment are always accompanied by compassion.[91] The classic texts in the Hebrew Scriptures, especially Second and Third Isaiah, speak loudly of a time of restoration and universal harmony.

One finds this synthesis of forecasting doom yet hoping for a peaceful resolution to forestall it in contemporary prophets as well. Malcolm X spent most of his life fueled by disdain of white America over its racist construction of a virtually unclimbable pyramid of inequality; what Dubois called a "a 'manure' theory of social organization."[92] However, after making the *Hajj* to Mecca, he experienced a conversion as he viewed white and black Muslims from around the world praying side by side without a hint of discrimination. He was grilled by sarcastic reporters in an airport news conference upon returning to New York about his "Letter from Mecca." He stated: "My pilgrimage broadened my scope. It blessed me with a new insight … In the past, yes, I have made sweeping indictments of *all* white people. I will never be guilty of that again."[93]

Even George Jackson, despite the tragic and violent events at the end of his imprisonment, often wrote in measured terms of respect for his adversaries and for a world of peace and unity:

> At each phase of the long train of tyrannies, we have conducted ourselves in a very meek and civilized manner, with only polite pleas for justice and moderation, all to no avail … We have remonstrated,

supplicated, demonstrated, and prostrated ourselves at the feet of our self-appointed administrators. We have done all that we can do to circumvent the eruption that now comes on apace.[94]

Coda

We have provided a set of traits that exemplify the life and message of the prophets: the lessons they deliver are discomforting and unwanted; they stand steadfastly with those incidental or threatening to the comfortable and powerful; they live in solitude and anguish; they are mentally unstable; and they are the bearers of an ultimately compassionate message. If we were to seek a common thread that links these qualities with the harassment and persecution they so often receive, the tie that binds them would be their estrangement from prevailing notions of common sense.

Common sense

Common sense refers to those ideas and conventions that any particular social configuration recognizes as patently truthful or morally good. It is a congeries of sacrosanct and unquestioned facts. Skinner claims that it is what group members "find reinforcing" due to "their genetic endowment and the natural and social contingencies to which they have been exposed."[95] It complements science in that while the latter seeks to elucidate universal truths, the maxims of common sense are largely addressed to particular matters. Put another way, science seeks to explicate the relation of things to one another, while common sense concerns itself with their relation to us.[96]

The power of common sense, according to Weber, is found in its association with the comfort lodged in "the sanctity of everyday routines."[97] More substantively, it provides the groundwork for initial steps in cognitive formulations. Its domain is "literal knowledge," what Langer calls the "the abstracted conception of things" and that to which those things stand in association. It does not dig into the terrain of intellectual elaboration. Rather, its conclusions are ready at hand, prompt, and categorical.[98] In Lonergan's phraseology, it evidences the credo that "knowing is like looking."[99]

This sensible and orderly canopy spread over everyday affairs and communicative patterns is, for Wittgenstein, the "halo" that surrounds thought and, in an echo of Kierkegaard, creates the order of "possibilities."[100] He contends that most of us believe that publicly accepted truths do not tread beyond the enclosure set by the empirical; they must be located in objective reality "for we think we already see [them] there."[101] The upshot is that one's secure "mental state" and the postulates that effortlessly spring from it, while not guaranteeing what will take place in the future, easily summon the conclusion in the here and now that one cannot conceive "where a doubt could get a foothold nor where a further test [is] possible."[102] Schopenhauer likewise posits the halo effect of common sense. For within its capsulized horizon, the motives and aims by which persons measure their conduct and that of others enable them to always provide a coherent account of specific ideas and actions. However, he states that if such persons were to be interrogated as to why they willed in such a way, they "would have no answer."[103]

This construct imposed upon naked experience provides a shield of psychic protection held by the institutional order with its ability to shelter the average citizen from the tempest of necessity and "madness." This is but an echo of Schutz's concept of the "natural attitude." Within its confines, a smooth surface of stability is maintained that, although ephemeral, gives every indication that the plans of "this-worldly realists" are securely grounded and their fulfillment confidently expected. It is part and parcel of common sense that it, like the natural attitude, fastens upon barriers against whim, chance, and the inexplicable. The natural attitude is "in the first place not an object of our thought but a field of domination." It conveys the "necessity of complying with the basic requirements of our life" and, consequently, in both an actual and potential sense, the objects it fastens upon as "primarily important" are or will become "ends or means for the realization of my projects."[104] It brackets any form of "doubt that the world and its objects might be otherwise" than what they appear to be.[105]

In Hegel's schema, the person employing common sense relies upon feeling, upon "an oracle in his breast, he is finished and done with anyone who does not agree."[106]

From a psychiatric perspective, Gillet states that persons ineluctably latch onto "techniques that are informal and subjective" through engaging in situations and relationships where "linguistic terms or signs mark certain ways of responding to the world." From repeated encounters, common sense, what is performatively normative or "sane" (here remembering Erving Goffman), permeates one's view of reality and "the actual world of human discourse." It establishes a corresponding and useful set of cognitive skills affecting individual functioning. Thus, the logical and coherent thinker learns to shape her use of concepts "according to the normative reactions of others to her judgments."[107]

Kant's philosophy takes Gillet and Goffman a step further, anchoring the power of common sense to shape intellectual and moral responses within the categorical imperative (a set of binding, rationally available mandates that are universal in scope and consequence).

Kant centers on a key ingredient of common sense: it, like morality, finds its basis, authenticity, and binding power in human reason. It is related to sensation and its propensity to judge—he uses the word "taste" to depict this—for it tends to function according to "a certain rule that I represent as valid for everyone." However, the experiential phenomenon itself cannot make a claim of universality. This can only be accomplished by what he calls "appreciative taste" that has an *a priori* foundation enabling it to transcend the pleasure I may receive in a particular object and provide it with transcendent validity.[108] This satisfaction that I may feel regarding the meaning of certain phenomena has no warrant until it produces a sense of clarity and truthfulness that gains its power to bind because it signifies an agreement of my affirmation "with the feeling of everyone else according to a universal law and so from reason."[109]

Of presiding interest for our purposes, Kant writes that the inner sense is logically subjective and therefore "subject to *illusions*." Thus, it can either mistake what is perceived internally as "actually happening outwardly" or, "equally erroneous," one might believe "that one is experiencing an actual inner revelation caused by another being that is not an object of outer sense." Both are illusions that trick us and, in each case, "we are dealing with *mental illness*."[110]

Kant therefore provides at the end of the eighteenth century, a convincing justification for a course of repressive action against those inwardly convinced of a message from the depths of their being.

A current psychiatric manual establishes its commonsense logic by sailing in the strong current driven by Kant's conclusions. The author writes that "peculiar motor behaviors" such as grimacing and abnormal movement "make your patient stand out, as social norms (or rules of common sense) are violated without obvious reason." He further adds that such symptoms, abetted by "delusions" and "clear cut hallucinations" are evidence of "psychosis" in that they are not only "held with great conviction even in the face of overwhelming evidence to the contrary" but also "are not shared by members of the patient's own culture or subculture."[111]

History has proven repeatedly the depiction of Kant and those influenced by him that madness is a belief in both the reality and validity of subjective inner experience. Nor has that history halted the confident, and largely unchallenged, determinations of psychiatric experts that such encounters are proof of psychosis and, in many cases, provide the *coup de grâce* that severs the relation between the visionary and free society. Foucault, once again, puts an exclamation point on the process in its justification of a "uniform world of exclusion." Gone is the earlier belief that subliminal and extra-empirical encounters constituted a "sign of another world." Rather, such experiences became a "manifestation of nonbeing ... Confinement is the practice which corresponds most exactly to madness experienced as unreason."[112]

Critique of common sense

There can be no argument that at the individual level, common sense is useful and essential to basic human interaction in a host of ways. It provides a vital service in socialization to shared norms and functions. It can serve to constrain prejudice as well as tendencies inimical to public welfare. Also, as Rowan Williams wisely reflects, since language is never static, it can generate "new possibilities of performance" that "add to the cumulative sum of adopted strategies." In this way, conventional discourse can open itself to possibilities "beyond the realm of specific causal processes."[113]

However respectable and noteworthy its virtues may be at the personal and social level, as a group phenomenon, common sense is often reactionary to new ideas and prone to a bias against cultural and religious minorities.[114] This engrained intolerance is what Lonergan refers to as scotosis: "an aberration of understanding" that fails to attend to insights and, moreover, meets them with inhibition and resistance.[115] His words amplify the way the mentally "aberrant" have regularly been dismissed both from our collective psyche and our social milieu. He states that the "general bias of common sense" is never far from "the notion that only ideas backed by some sort of force can be operative."[116]

The intellectual and moral formulations of common sense are incapable of referencing or being significantly influenced by history writ large or, often, by the persecution of currently targeted "out groups," writ small. A sensitivity to the lessons of history or to hermeneutical reformulation is far removed from what Lonergan calls "the scotosis of the dramatic subject" or the prejudicial responses of dominant groups "that realize only the ideas they see to be to their immediate advantage." This pragmatism, this sense of the immediacy of generally accepted behavioral nostrums, is foreign to taking a long view of the development of ideas and social formulae. Such a resistance to "higher integrations" means that it must take a blunt force approach to "intricate and disputed issues," say, for instance, those raised then and now by the prophet.[117]

In much the same way that scientific paradigms condition the way new information is processed and investigative inquiries carried out, common sense is incapable, on its own legs, to bear the weight of ideological interjections that threaten its conclusions. This in spite of the fact that what is inherited in shared discourse consists of not only "sound ideas but also incomplete ideas, mutilated ideas, enthusiasms, passions, [and] bitter memories."[118]

The sociology of knowledge then comes into play with its webs of thought, shielded by the assurance that those on the periphery of true discourse, those labeled incoherent compared to the way "sane" people talk and communicate, are deranged and sanction worthy. To reference Leo Strauss, the "uncanny" nature of prophetic utterances is viewed "as the height of danger."[119]

To sum up this critique, the bias inherent in common sense cannot be rectified by common sense.[120] Its formulations are incomplete until complemented by ideas emanating from outside the realm of the practical and the particular. It stands in need of intrepid or desperate souls who stand their ground against the onslaught of inertia, social conservatism, and prejudicial bias.

The rationalism lauded by the purveyors of order and norm and by the medical materialist, revealed in the truncated paths to security and self-development in a meritocratic hierarchy, is deaf to accounts of human flourishing and conclusions unknown to conventional pedagogy and scientific certainty. Witness the logic of Fingarette: "We say of a person who is insane that he is irrational. When he manifests his insanity in his conduct, it is natural to speak of his conduct as irrational. An insane person has 'lost his reason'."[121]

Such right brain bias fails to convince or convert those attending to deeper sources of knowledge and conviction. In fact, William James states categorically that if "you have intuitions at all, they come from a deeper level of your nature." The interior life, the life of faith, the inspirations of subconscious revelation continually surface convincing premises and the person acclimatized to the winds of the spirit "feels the weight of the result." As we have broached so often in our study, something within "absolutely *knows* that that result must be truer than any logic-chopping rationalistic talk, however clever, that may contradict it."[122]

Insight

Recall Kierkegaard's contention that depression is universal. Few can weather the tensions created by an open-eyed appraisal of life's precarious stability; its tragic, and often fatal, calamities; and the temptation either to live in denial or succumb to what earlier prognoses of mental handicaps call melancholia. Only the latter assembly can find release and serenity in a leap of faith. It is in the throes of uncertainty and openness to a light shining within that uncommon revelations and insights are perceived. Foucault is correct in his appraisal and appreciation of that dynamic state and its counterintuitive conclusions. He speaks of an inner connection

> which permits the sufferer to predict the future, to speak in an unknown language, to see beings ordinarily invisible; this melancholia originates in a supernatural intervention, the same which brings to the sleeper's mind those dreams which foresee the future, announce events to come, and cause him to see "strange things."[123]

As with the critique of common sense, I will base much of the exposition on insight upon the ideas of Bernard Lonergan aided by an array of noted scholars.

For Lonergan, the nature of insight is closely related to the typology developed by William James to describe mystical encounters to which we alluded previously. For James, in such transformative moments the recipient does not conjure the event, he or she is entirely passive; the occurrence is indescribable in empirical or positivist terms (ineffable); it imparts a concrete, noetic message; and it is short in duration.[124] In Lonergan's portrayal, insight comes "as release to the tension of inquiry"; it comes "suddenly and unexpectedly"; it derives not from "outer circumstances but inner conditions"; it stands in the tension "between the concrete and the abstract"; "it passes into the habitual texture of one's mind," and it implies a metaphysics.[125]

Let us look more closely at the characteristics of insight just provided.

Insight is uncanny and unwanted

A classic instance of the adverse reaction caused by insight is found in the Gospel of Luke with the memorable words of Jesus that "no prophet is accepted" (Lk. 4:24). He had come to the synagogue in his hometown and had accompanied this claim with words that so infuriated his former friends and neighbors that they drove him to the brink of the cliff upon which the town was built with the intention of killing him. He had said that God looked more favorably upon a widow from Sidon (in present-day Lebanon) at the time of Elijah the prophet than those in Israel; he then upped the ante by claiming that of the many lepers alive in the time of Elisha the prophet, none received healing from God, via Elisha, save a commander of the Syrian army, an archenemy of the Jewish people, who had forced a captive Israelite woman into his servitude (Lk. 4:25–29).

This evocative story serves to underscore Lonergan's claim that insights, such as those offered by the prophets, are unwelcome precisely because they seek to overturn and revise the secure and self-assured point of view condoned by common accord.[126] Their genesis in the imagination places them, by definition, far from the constraints set by day to day, conventional speech and, more to the point, the solution to their dissemination is normally some form of repression.[127] Wittgenstein corroborates this observation with his contention that what we are terming insight is perceived by those threatened by its dictates as nonsense. Yet, he claims that what is banned as senseless does not necessarily lack a coherent thought pattern. Rather, it is communicated with a combination of words that have been "excluded from the language, withdrawn from circulation."[128]

Wittgenstein enlarges his perspective with reference to his influential concept of "language games." He argues that what is commonly denoted as "fitting" or understandable is far more complicated than its supporters might recognize. Those logical constructions are no more than a game played with words whose parameters have the appearance of solidity and inviolability that often summons retaliation when regularized social and moral meanings are confronted by new definitions of human worth and ethical conduct.[129] Indeed, language-games thrive not on reconciling diverse viewpoints but by comparing the innovative with what is conventionally true.[130]

To be considered an insight, any new social or moral construction must, by definition, be creative. What it introduces, citing Whitehead, is novelty. And that novelty, as with prophetic parlance, moves invariably from the "disjunctive" to the "conjunctive"; from difference, separation, and antagonism to coherence, community, and harmony.[131] That predilection for overcoming boundaries, however, is rarely affirmed by those circumscribed by narrowly defined limits of language and action. As Rieff claims, the formulations of scientific investigation normally lack the capacity to develop the "ardent imaginations necessary to the forming of new communities."[132] Despite the interpersonal accord required to maintain the ethical and social tenets of common sense, its map of acceptable variation, its social geography is not one of inclusivity but exclusion. It features the gutting of a general sense of incorporating the extraneous to one that is suspicious of difference. Jock Young asks: "Are we heading toward a dystopia of exclusion, where division occurs not only between nations ... but within the nations themselves? Can one part of a room remain forever warm whilst the other half is perpetually closed off and cold?" He argues that this state of affairs now has the ring of inevitability "and forms a functioning, if oppressive, whole."[133]

Insight involves a sudden release from inner tension

From Heschel's perspective, insight is the result of "much intellectual dismantling and dislocation." The prophets about whom he writes are facing significant mental and emotional strain. They are the recipients of feelings and suspicions that are "unfamiliar, unparalleled, incredible" that constitute a breakthrough. Insight then reveals "a way of seeing the phenomenon from within." It is surprising and "entails genuine perception." The inner churning, as it were, produces what he calls "knowledge at first sight."[134]

He is referring to an elementary knowing whose efficient cause is the data received through experience, yet to know in a fully human way, the conceptual vocabulary provided by experience initially raises many more questions and doubts than it does conclusions. Those unsettling objections are, for Lonergan, "the catalyst for the genesis of insight."[135]

I am reminded here of the case of Joseph M. Giarratano. A convicted murderer arrested in 1979, he was condemned to death for the crime. His appeal, however, which surfaced a host of procedural judicial errors, led the governor of Virginia at that time to commute his sentence in 1991 to imprisonment for life. The disturbing circumstances surrounding his trial led Giarratano to a deliberate and detailed study of law. At first his motivation was solely to petition for DNA testing and a possible retrial (he was finally granted parole in 2017). However, the questions about which Heschel and Lonergan speak led to an unveiling of a previously unknown reality. As a result, he undertook to direct his newfound legal knowledge and considerable intellectual acumen (one of his monographs was published in the *Yale Law Review*) to establish programs on nonviolent activism as well as to take on the cases of other lifers in their quest for a remission of sentence due to extenuating circumstances or alleged judicial oversight. As a result of his intra-institutional efforts, he was transferred to a prison in Utah and subsequently placed in one of Virginia's two supermax penitentiaries, his personality having been determined to be mired in actual as well as potential mischief.[136]

This serves as a telling example of prophetic inspiration received as a clarity that releases the recipient of inner turmoil. Lonergan doubts whether "any specialists in the field of psychiatry" have the disciplinary resources to link the kind of insight just spoken of with both intellectual illumination and psychic renewal and recovery.[137]

Insight derives from inner conditions

Among the themes in her well-regarded volume, *The Fragility of Goodness*, Martha Nussbaum ponders the way prophecy and insight are foregrounded in classic Greek texts, such as the "Phaedrus" by Plato. In her analysis of the discussion of love in that dialogue, she writes of the knowledge that lovers gain in that exalted state. She concludes that aside from the readily observable effects and commitments, love surfaces an "intuitive understanding of how to act ... how to teach, how to respond, how to limit oneself." For Socrates, such inner direction "is insight," one that is "crucial to moral and intellectual development."[138]

Lonergan reprieves this hidden knowledge and its birth in an inner cauldron of primeval passions and noetic conviction. Like Nussbaum, he speaks of the observable or empirical "knowns" in experience that can be apprehended as sense data, the "unknowns ... are what one will grasp by insight." The resulting "conceptions and suppositions" from this mysterious source are far more than subjective inklings, they reveal the very nature of reality.[139]

Continuing this thought pattern, insight is attained not by conscious deduction, nor by "learning rules," nor "by following precepts," nor "by studying any methodology." What the seer, prophet, or mystic receives is a new beginning, a set of "new rules that supplement or even supplant the old." Theirs is creative genius in that it not only "disregards established routines," it announces the new ideas and practices "that will be the routines of the future."[140]

The knowledge of the positivist or ardent pragmatist works within intellectual limits determined by external phenomena. In this, the poverty of empirical experience is manifested. However, the capacity of thought transcends the empirical for, as we have noted repeatedly, the boundaries of cognition are set from within "by the power of conception, the wealth of formulative notions with which the mind meets experience." Langer reminds us that the novel and creative are surfaced by those capable of seeing things hidden in plain sight.[141]

A prisoner's reflection addresses this multi-layered nature of wisdom and understanding. The author claims that it is based upon the insight that "knowledge derived from the senses is illusory; true knowledge can only come from the understanding of the union of opposites." He writes, citing an ancient alchemical text, that what is above and what is below must be brought into harmony: "as above, so below; as below, so above."[142] It is reminiscent of St. Paul's words in Ephesians (1:8–10): "God has given us the wisdom to understand fully the mystery … to bring all things into one … in the heavens and on earth."

This attunement of a state of wonder to insights welling up from the subconscious was, as we have spoken of so often, a preoccupation of William James, particularly regarding those stigmatized as psychologically pathological. The ones affected by "crankiness, insane temperament, loss of mental balance, [and] psychopathic degeneration" possess a particular temperament that "when combined with a superior quality of intellect, in an individual, make it more probable that he will make his mark and affect his age."[143] Of course, the proximate effect, as we have seen with notable figures, and less notable "geniuses," may well be claustration in a prison cell.

Insight is concrete and abstract

As mentioned earlier, insight is intentionally directed to real-life affairs, but its source in the secret portals of the unconscious is ultimately unknowable. Whitehead captures the essence of this union of the noumenal and the phenomenal in noting that insight is grounded in first principles, far beyond the range of the analytical mind. We spoke in Chapter 2 of the "deficiencies of language" that lie at the root of tensions between worldviews. While Whitehead would concur with our thesis that there is no first principle that cannot be encountered "by a flash of insight" and provide some noetic assurance, the very limitations of language and "imaginative penetration" forbid any simple formulation that can be grasped by those outside the experience providing the revelation.[144]

This takes us back to our thoughts regarding Jung and the archetypal images and energies that connect us to what he believes are the basic truths of existence.[145] Facing both the personal and collective qualities of these primal messages, brings to us "the very undeveloped archaic energy" of insights, instinctual urges, and powerful desires and "force[s] them into consciousness." Thinking of the reluctance of the emissary prophet, the "archaic force" propels the recipient to direct energy to collective crises and distorted values from a hidden and alien conceptual arsenal. He or she indeed shudders before the *massa confusa*, yet through such "threatening spiritual visions" the new comes in.[146]

Lonergan states that the territory of insight is not crossed in charting the relations between data but in finding and grasping the unity, the identity, the "whole in data," in blending the particular and the abstract "in their totality of aspects."[147]

In reference to our study, we have been arguing that many schizophrenics, usually the poor, the homeless, and those perceived to be threatening or troublesome, are the recipients of internal messages and visons that reveal a heterogeneity of influences unknowable and, ultimately, intolerable in a fact-based, materialist world. As Sass correctly surmises, to this reductionist ideology, "almost any generalization one applies to such patients will seem, on further consideration, almost counter to the truth."[148]

Insight becomes part of the mind's habitual structure

As a phenomenologist, Schutz posited that what can be known, can only be grasped in the bracketing of our subjective thoughts and feelings about a person, an object, or an experience and entering into relation with it in an atmosphere of care and acceptance. In this approach to life, "the world in no way vanishes from the field of experience," rather what is grasped "is the pure life of consciousness in which and through which the whole objective world exists for me."[149]

Thinking back to one of Schutz's intellectual mentors, Edmund Husserl, there is "an infinitude of knowledge, previous to all deduction."[150] In the effort to empty the ego of its need to relate all to itself and judge each person and thing accordingly, one finds, in that emptiness, a stable world of transcendent ideas, unreachable to those trapped in self-preoccupation. As Husserl claims, the residue of this dying to oneself is an "*apriori*" composed of "indissoluble essential structures of transcendental subjectivity, which persist in and through all imaginable modifications."[151] In this, we have yet another lens with which to view the people whose experiences of the noumenal, so tantalizingly real for them, find themselves in a world deaf and blind to what is, literally, before their ears and eyes.

Wittgenstein comes up with a similar conclusion (shorn of transcendent inferences) that privileges ineluctable internal notions of veracity: "I did not get my picture of the world by satisfying myself of its correctness ... No: it is the inherited background against which I distinguish between true and false." It is the product of a system in which all hypotheses about the real find their foundation and justification. It is "the element in which arguments have their life."[152]

Once insights are embraced, we arrive at a place, "a supreme moment," when all that we see merges into a single perspective. At that point, indicative of the prophet, "sweeping yet accurate deductions become possible, and subsequent exact predictions regularly will prove to have been correct."[153] To the chagrin of those who must bear the presence of the prophetic, the entire established order of knowledge is thrown into reverse. Of course, the real and the apparent exist for both but their evaluative context is radically disparate. For the prophet, unlike her troubled neighbor, what is empirically real recedes to the realm of the microscopic, while what is the "merely apparent" becomes macroscopic in which basic truths are inerrantly verified.[154]

One long-time prisoner reveals how "despair and loneliness" eventually led to "significant insight." For example, in sharing how prison is "an abyss set to diminish you from within," he states that when confronted with the often heartbreaking and mind-numbing experience of solitary confinement, he learned to discover the benefits to be found in such solitude: "quiet time, exercise, reading a good book with no distractions … and a sort of time out from the environment that stops you from seeing the bigger picture."[155] His narrative echoes the thoughts of Lonergan who claims that in the optimal framework for the reception of insight, the "interests and hopes, desires and fears, of ordinary living have to slip into the background." What surfaces, in the "detached and disinterested" inner vacuum is a new mode of seeing and acquiring intelligence.[156]

This dynamic interrelation between the observable and the intuitive, as Gillet reports, clarifies one's place and conduct in the world as well as one's thoughts about the world. It smoothly integrates them into a self-revelatory viewpoint: "When I attain knowledge congruent with that ideal, I am said to have *insight* into my condition as a human being."[157]

Insight implies a metaphysics

To have insight into insight implies a metaphysics.[158] Our discussion of the prophetic in this chapter has alerted us to the resounding fact that the prophet does not follow the academic ritual of hypothesis, research, writing, and, ideally, publication. The "goodness" of the prophets is not the result of disseminating pieces of knowledge to be ruminated upon by their peers. Goodness in this sense is an engagement with what is believed to be the source of the good; it is a mysterious but nonetheless real relationship with forces that far surpass common sense or the logical canons prescribed to validate a supposition. As Cassirer relates, the mission of the prophets and the content of their pronouncements are the result of "direct spiritual insight." Their conviction of the righteousness and authenticity of their activity and what it intends to communicate is itself the result of a communication breathed from their very soul. What makes them alternately so compelling and shocking is their belief that "they have been given a special insight into the mind of God."[159]

The prophet fulfills the basic definition of transcendence in always "going beyond" the first formulations of knowledge and perception and engaging in "the elementary matter of raising further questions."[160] This accompanies an ontological claim of the indivisibility of matter and spirit in humans just as in "electrons and atoms, plants and animals."[161]

We have focused throughout this volume on the traditional metaphysical themes of being and unity. What is revealed as a result of that focus necessarily involves the intellect and its relation to being and the interrelation of all forms of matter. This intelligibility, as Lonergan claims (and as we have observed repeatedly regarding the subjects of our study), can be scientific in reference to the empirical but it can also be constrained by that very condition. In contrast, however, "spiritual intelligibility is comprehensive; its reach is the universe of being; and it is in virtue of that reach not only that [one] can know the universe but also that the universe can bring forth its own unity in the concentrated form of a single intelligent view."[162]

Conclusion

We have probed in this chapter the inner tension, the cross of conviction, and the mysterious receptivity of the prophet, paraphrasing Spinoza, to the One who wrote all. It is a lonely vocation, unbearable in many instances, yet one preternaturally essential if the giver of life is to save creature and creation from the obscene debasement they have suffered and continue to suffer. For we have all, to varying degrees, dared to eat from the tree of the knowledge of good and evil and, in so doing, have sought to usurp dominion over who is sane and insane, who is worthy and unworthy of basic human care, and who should live and who should die. Some among us, however fragile, must challenge this death march. How could a task be more ominous, more frightening, and more indispensable?

We have attempted a character analysis of these chosen souls and, in a more formulaic manner, viewed their task in reference to common sense and insight. One thing is clear: the message of prophets true to the name cannot be tolerated, whether they are rebellious agitators or homeless people sleeping in the subway. It is to the distinction between those two expressions that we now turn.

5

Prophetic Types and the Penal Sanctuary

We have spoken repeatedly of prophets in these pages in both their voluntary and involuntary guises. In this chapter we will elaborate upon these two expressions. We will first speak of the voluntary prophets and their radical ministrations against skewed opportunity and the detention of the threatening in a culture dominated by the fear, projection, and victimization of its "partial citizens" and "internal exiles." Since, in the last chapter, our profile of the prophetic character was largely a synopsis of the voluntary prophet, our remarks in this area will be rather brief and amplify the courageous witness of some imprisoned prophets. We will then proceed to analyze the involuntary prophets whose inability to bear the heavy cloak of necessity, as alluded to in our discussion of Kierkegaard, so often creates an alternate reality that is as much colored by internal/religious intimations as it is by fanciful illusion. That exposition will then be followed by discussing a synonym for the prison that, by now, should strike the reader as most apropos. More and more, our detention facilities have become the sanctuaries of the prophets.

The voluntary prophet: determination to speak the truth despite fierce opposition

There are those in this world who are blessed and burdened with a deep sensitivity to issues pertaining to justice, fairness, and equal regard, particularly for those whose lives are in daily peril. Furthermore, they are moved by an unknown force to relinquish their reluctance to sacrifice personal desires for security and comfort, even to cling tenaciously to their very lives, in fidelity to what can be depicted in no other way than an inner fire. This prophetic flame cannot be quenched unless the appointed person speaks and acts on behalf of those whose immeasurable worth has been distorted and whose lives are perceived to possess no social value. Such persons are what I am calling voluntary prophets. As Brueggemann attests, they resist "totalism": those systemic practices and constraints that seek to eliminate critical retort or intrusion. They are, as we discussed in the last chapter, inevitably at the very edge of the "inside," in the ghettos and jails from which they find a ground "to think the unthinkable, to imagine the unimaginable, and to utter the unutterable."[1]

Such a determined and reluctant prophet is Mohamedou Ould Slahi, an engineer from Mauritania, educated in Germany, who was arrested in 2001 on the suspicion that he was one of the architects of the plot to blow up the World Trade Center in New York. He was held captive in several interrogation camps before being transferred to Guantanamo Bay, Cuba, where he was subjected to various forms of physical and psychological abuse until his release in 2016. While impounded in a secret prison in Jordan, he was made to walk blindfolded past the torture room where he could hear the screams. On Guantanamo, one of the ordeals he faced was to endure what his captors called "the recipe." His books, including the Koran, were taken from him and he was placed in a box: "The ... box was cooled down to where I was shaking most of the time. I was forbidden from seeing the light of day ... For the next seventy days I wouldn't know the sweetness of sleeping: interrogation twenty-four hours a day."[2] His response to his tormentors and their threats and acts of violence reveals the strength given to some courageous souls to witness to the truth in spite of all obstacles: "You don't know me. I swear by Almighty God I'll never talk to you. Go ahead and torture me. It will take my death to make me talk."[3]

Another intrepid survivor of torture, in this instance in the Soviet Gulag, was Taras Shevshenko. Writing about his tribulation some years later he reveals that "not a single lineament in my inner self has changed. I thank my Creator with all my heart and soul that He has not allowed my horrible experience to touch my beliefs with its iron claws."[4]

Resistance to persecutors convinced of a captive's guilt only feeds bloodlust and the frenzy that erupts from a disfigured spirit with unrestricted power over the other, as Slahi among so many others have given painful witness.

Solzhenitsyn experienced this unbridled cruelty and saw it ruthlessly applied on too many occasions:

> That was why they felt no mercy, but, instead, an explosion of resentment and rage toward those maliciously stubborn prisoners who opposed being fitted into the totals, who would not capitulate to sleeplessness or the punishment cell or hunger. By refusing to confess they menaced the interrogator's personal standing ... In such circumstances all measures were justified![5]

Solzhenitsyn is surely a prophet in his courageous denunciation of the brutality of the Soviet regime. His own survival was often at peril. Yet, he attributes his ability to endure the crushing time in confinement to the solace provided by a crudely constructed rosary. He had noticed the Catholic Lithuanian prisoners making rosaries by soaking pieces of bread. These fellow sufferers, touched by his religious devotion, "with true brotherly love," helped him assemble one of his own. He had to hide it inside his mittens, which were wide enough to enable him to finger the beads unnoticed, especially when passing through checkpoints. Solzhenitsyn states unequivocally that "this necklace helped me to write and remember."[6]

An imprisoned Muslim, this time in a prison in Georgia, is Hamim Abdullah Muadh-Dhin Asadallah, dubbed by his captors as "the white Martin Luther King." He helped coordinate a labor strike among those forced to work as a way of pressuring the administration to provide for the workers a living wage, access to education, decent health care, healthy nutrition, and a respectful human environment. He was beaten by three White correctional officers "because of the prison strike, my religion ... and because of my love for all Black people" and subsequently placed in solitary confinement for months. From there, he crafted a letter seeking support from human rights leaders and organizations. His appeal found its stark answer in his being placed in a cell with no bed where he was left naked, deprived of food and prescription medication for two days.[7] Yet he remains undaunted in his public witness on behalf of his imprisoned brothers.

A prisoner currently serving time in California captures the essence of the rage felt by "a massive and bitterly angry underclass" as well as the prophet's reminder that such abuse will bring catastrophic repercussions:

> And make no mistake about it, no one who experiences this system, whether as a prisoner or the loved one or friend of a prisoner, is not angry and bitter. The system, which defines itself as society's protector, as the bulwark against chaos and anarchy, is sowing the seeds of society's destruction.[8]

What drives such passionate responses to human degradation? As mentioned previously, voluntary prophets somehow believe that it is worth what many would judge a futile effort to resist the tide of injustice while, almost inevitably, being borne within its destructive current, sometimes to their own deaths. The prophet has hope, perhaps not for herself, but for the righteousness of the cause; or that God, or the echo of the moral goodness lying in the inner sanctum of her hearers, will motivate them to turn from their reticence, intransigence, or rancor and lead them to a change of heart.

There is a madness here. One that sees beyond the conflict, the rejection, the threats to personal safety, and the massive negation of the sacredness of so many lives. As de Young writes, whether bestowed upon "the Holy Fool, the mad artist, the wild-eyed prophet or the insane genius," what many term to be madness becomes the avenue through which "prophecy, creativity, inspiration, insight, and even love" are engendered and communicated despite the cost.[9]

Rudolf Otto recognizes the rarity and singular importance of such an exceptional acuity. He states that most of us indeed have a "predisposition," a general susceptibility to acknowledge the basic moral and spiritual truths of religion out of our native psychic capacity. This, however, is contrasted with the "Spirit" which takes on a universal perceptiveness and sensitivity in the form of "*testimonium Spiritus internum*" (internal spiritual testimony). This elevated stage is "a sphere of religion" inhabited by "*the prophet.*" Otto contends that the prophet is the mirror in the spiritual plane of the creative artist, the one in "whom the Spirit shows itself alike as the power to hear the 'voice'" and "the power of divination."[10]

The revelations of voluntary prophets, paraphrasing one prisoner, do not simply drop into their laps, but, as Otto suggests, are in the domain of the mystical, the imaginative, and the poetic. In that "spiritual climate necessary for the attainment of meaning," the prophets transmit to the "sensory world" its disguised or deflected meaning. The hearers, if able to sweep away the cobwebs and ideological blinders distorting their vision can then consider "what seems to be a meaningless life and universe" are filled with "deeper truths that are life affirming."[11]

Relating voluntary prophecy back to the label of insanity, Laing states that when a person is perceived to experience madness, "a profound transposition of his place in relation to all domains of being occurs." As noted regarding schizophrenia, the center of experience moves from the egoic or outward self and goes inward to the much deeper instinctual dimensions of the imagination and the unconscious. Reminiscent of St. Augustine's understanding of time, chronological time "becomes merely anecdotal, only the eternal matters." This latter state is timeless. The two are blended in the "mad" person who conflates the ego and the deeper self, the outer and inner worlds, the natural and the supernatural. Laing suggests that despite the "profound wretchedness and degradation" that one regularly experiences in this bi-dimensional existence, he or she becomes a hierophant or interpreter of the eternal. Although he may have lost his sense of place in the world, "we are distracted from our cozy security by this mad ghost who haunts us with … visions and voices which seem so senseless and of which we feel impelled to rid him, cleanse him, cure him."[12]

In summary, the voluntary prophet is rooted in the contingency of the human condition, knows pain, loss, and renunciation, yet is given the courage and insight to feel and express dissatisfaction with a fractured world. Remembering Heidegger, he or she is "thrown" into an encounter with Being, either by an explicit act of faith such as that exhibited by Slahi and Solzhenitsyn, or simply by the stirrings and subtle messages from an inner source.[13] She comes to see the "radical deficiency" in every concrete expression of the world in which she resides. As Jaspers surmises, the prophet is nourished by "another root of his Being than that of his finiteness."[14]

The involuntary prophet: diffuse rage over social injustice

As has been mentioned often, I include among the involuntary prophets those persons categorized as mentally ill whose comportment is predicated largely on their disjointed attempts to face their own spiritual, psychological, and social alienation with unblinking fortitude. Recall the predominance of the schizophrenic label appended to people dwelling in the inner-city slums and ghettos of America, Great Britain, and elsewhere. We have argued that the designation is a convenient justification to apply the psychotic label with its accompanying stigmata of alarm, intolerance, and banishment.

The stigmata, of course, contain a level of truth. Remembering Kierkegaard, the attempt to reconcile the inner and outer worlds, heavily dependent on the intimations, revelations, and insights of the former, do indeed verify the presence of "nervous disorders." For, as the philosopher acknowledges, one avoids the despair of those unaware of their despair, only to succumb to the burden of finitude and, often, inner disclosures that, like the victims of torture whose stories we just narrated, drive the spirit to a brink of nothingness that can only be bridged by faith.[15] As we know, these celestial or imaginative visons have mobilized the culture at large and the medical and judicial community, in particular, to cart into social oblivion so many attuned to such insightful or hallucinatory encounters.

We made much in the last two chapters of the realistic grasp of these prophets. This awareness is triggered by an inner light that illumines, albeit in inchoate ways, the inequities of the economic system and the all-seeing eyes and ravenous jaws of the security and law enforcement complex. These forces, for their part, allow them no escape from their unstable lives, their meagre standard of living, their frequent homelessness, and, just as frequently, the sting of handcuffs and a hard seat on the bus to the local house of detention. We sought to upend the sanity hierarchy by stressing that the wake for their "social death" and their cultural burial unleashes the possibility of a resurrected faith. Moreover, their demotion to the lowest rung on the success ladder also summons intimations and messages from the wellspring of creativity; one that arises from the "inability to accept the standard cultural denials of the real nature of experience."[16]

Yet, there is normally no sense, nor is one required, that the images through which they observe the world are indications of an honest confrontation with the reality of life's capriciousness, or that their rejection of facile social compromises laden with violence and deception are indeed prophetic. In other words, remembering Otto, the unsuspecting prophet requires no conscious "identification, in different degrees of completeness, of the personal self with the transcendent Reality."[17] She lives and is duly punished simply for witnessing in her awkward and perhaps incomprehensible utterances and gestures to the hypocrisy of trying to hide from the travails of naked existence behind the façade of normalcy. L. Mack Lendon, confined in Michigan, writes of his traumatic life and its penal finale that characterizes the attitude I am suggesting: "Am I a disgruntled prisoner? Of course I am. I had severe brain damage, been once left for dead, underwent brain surgery, been shot up, severely mentally ill, heavy substance abuser, and was repeatedly raped as a child. Damn right I'm disgruntled."[18]

William Fisher and his colleagues concur with this observation in adding that many among those susceptible to conditions such as schizophrenia engage in offensive actions or forms of deviant behavior not because they have a serious mental health problem but because they suffer due to the distressing conditions related to their poverty.[19]

In his sixth-century spiritual treatise, *The Ladder of Divine Ascent*, St. John Climacus gives a vivid description of a profound sorrow among penitent monks brought about by succumbing to life's tragic pitfalls that easily provokes acute mental distress:

> I saw there some who seemed from their demeanor to be out of their mind. In their great disconsolateness they had become like dumb men, in complete darkness, and were insensible to the whole of life. Their minds had already sunk to the very depths of humility, and they had burnt up the tears in their eyes with the fire of their despondency.[20]

While the disconsolateness described by St. John can lead to numbness and passivity, it can also trigger antisocial responses. In his study on the causes of such behavior, James Gilligan probes the tense relation between vivid experiences of personal and societal rejection and ensuing rage at the perpetrators of dehumanizing actions and the conditions that promote them. He asserts that one of the principal causes of this reactive conduct is found among the poor who are assaulted day after day in a society where human worth is regularly portrayed in the commercial and entertainment industries against the backdrop of material luxury and effortless social mobility. He writes that people are shamed vertically on a "systemic, wholesale basis" as populations are tiered according to in-groups and out-groups, the accepted and the neglected, the powerful and weak, the rich and the poor, and the mentally stable and unstable.[21] He elaborates further by concentrating on the perilous gap between one's personal aspirations for demonstrable rewards and what one, in fact, achieves.

In caste-dominated cultures, such as traditional Indian society, this divide is more easily weathered, particularly when interpreted in religious terms, as Louis Dumont pointed out some years ago.[22] In Western cultures, however, there is no intervening metaphysics that can deflect the feelings not only of inadequacy but also of a visceral sense of inferiority relative to more privileged sectors of the population. After all, the myth of equal opportunity not only inspires some; it also severely frustrates others. As Gilligan states, self-esteem is in many respects intrinsically woven to educational attainment, marketable skills, and socially respected and recognized achievements. Thus, "in the very materialist, capitalist culture in which we live," one's "net worth" is dramatically related to one's "self-worth." Poverty, lack of education, social immobility, and the jail cell that often awaits persons in those categories, fail to provide, in most instances, the compensatory psychological supports to weather feelings of anger and its accompanying effects.[23] Countless men and women have seen their life circumstances mocked and themselves marginalized under this omnipresent pressure.

Christopher Marshall views the resulting condition as "chronic shame." It emerges "when our ability to absorb or process shame is overwhelmed by its intensity or frequency, so that feelings of failure or unworthiness become a permanent state of being, a habitat in which the self is formed and operates."[24] He adds that socioeconomic position in a relentlessly competitive culture may be utilized "to mock or marginalize vulnerable groups, to project collective anxieties onto innocent scapegoats, to stigmatize those who differ from the majority in terms of appearance, belief, or identity, and to protect unjust power arrangements from challenge."[25]

This perplexing condition is reminiscent of David Nathanson's "compass of shame." Those reduced to inconsequentiality, the homeless for instance, are prone to emotional, if not physical withdrawal from contexts where shame might occur. As agents with their own inner barometer of psychic survival, they often "reject their rejectors" by self-aggrandizement or compulsive behaviors; they are frequently driven to self-harm or self-deprecation; and, as we have been suggesting, feel an animus against others fueled by rage over their ontological demotion.[26]

In the push and pull regarding intellectual handicaps and incarceration, this shame and rejection of rejectors is powerfully enforced. Barbara Harlow writes that the experience of detention "can, at given times and in particular circumstances, provide the historically necessary conjunctural premises" for reframing the narrative of justly deserved punishment as a subterfuge to dispose of sections of the population "by a sociopolitical system of economic exploitation and political disenfranchisement."[27]

Weber saw with his keen eye that the chances of garnering "social honor" are eliminated for those feeding on crumbs in the capitalist feast. Status and its accompanying rewards are predicated upon one's place in the meritocracy which, in turn, is typically associated with a "legally guaranteed and [legally] monopolized claim to sovereign rights or to income and profit."[28]

I am suggesting that the involuntary prophet, in his or her reactive anger at their disheartened condition and equally disheartening future, manifests the same divine displeasure with the way they and so many are condemned to a sordid half-life as animates the self-reflective political radical remonstrating against social injustice. Witness this ode concerning one just released from captivity: "Did a stretch in prison to be released to a cell. Returned to freedom penned by Orwell. My noon temptation is the Metro's third rail. In my wallet, I carry around my daguerreotype, A mugshot, no smiles, my name a tithe. What must I pay for being a stereotype?"[29]

Kierkegaard anticipates this adversity in pointing out that the powerless, the belittled, and the downtrodden are not "birds" who accept "naturally all that befalls [them]." They are well-aware of the distinctions that elevate some and debase others. The involuntary prophet or, in the former's terminology, "the knight of faith" knows and

> knows that others know … that he is a lowly human being, and he knows what this means. He knows also what is understood by the advantages of earthly life … and alas, that they are all denied to him … [T]hey seem to be for the purpose of indicating how lowly he is.

With every new advantage the eminent add to their eminence, the belittled one is forced to concede greater lowliness.[30]

The un-reflexive negative reaction to the world around her, coupled with her enforced and seemingly permanent diminutive status, leads easily into the sort of offenses that shuffle the "mentally ill" perpetrator into a jail cell. These actions fall into three categories: those who often commit "survival crimes"; those with antisocial tendencies exacerbated by the sort of mental strain we have so often described; and those who engage in violent behavior as a direct result of psychiatric symptoms.[31]

Such are the involuntary prophets: nameless, faceless, homeless; forgotten or simply ignored; yet animated by an inner reaction to their degradation and that of those dear to them that is birthed in the fire that created and sustains the universe. They are unwitting agents of that fire, but they are as stern and uncompromising in their disquieting presence as the most vocal and self-aware prophets of the past or present.

I am reminded of them in these words from the theologian, Hans Urs von Batlhasar:

Wholeness streams and shines through fragments … It is as if to renounce all efforts to achieve wholeness is precisely to practice wholeness itself, as if God is nowhere nearer than in the humility and poverty of indifference, in the openness to death, in the renunciation of every hold on or attempt to make certain of God.[32]

The prison as prophetic sanctuary

Throughout this volume, we have argued that criminal detention is more and more a euphemism for the removal of unwanted and bothersome elements of the general population. A host of factors have united to conspire both consciously and unconsciously to center that rejection upon the specter of madness, whether psychiatrically or socially determined, whether in the visage of the itinerant hordes sleeping on the streets, or in the angry voices calling and acting for a top to bottom reconstruction of economic and political policy.

The fact that incarceration and imprisonment have become the reflexive response to those we neither wish to see nor hear reveals personal and social pathologies among the "rejectors" that we have illuminated. It is worth noting how the very architecture that has become a metaphor for social deprivation itself contains a mirror for those pathologies. As Timothy Gorringe claims, the buildings in which people live shoulder a great deal of importance for we do not merely look at them, we "breathe them in." Architecture always concretizes a discourse, a manner of public address. At its worst, "it can be used to manipulate, as with Nazi stadiums, intending to overawe, or shopping malls, persuading us to buy."[33] The fact that we barely raise an eyebrow at the sight of a compound dressed in barbed wire does not lessen the way such "statements" involve and impact us. They are pockets of misery, pain, and violence that remind us of our explicit and implicit sanction of human denigration and the persecution of so many who reveal a truth we lack the ability or, perhaps, the courage to face.

From my perspective, this movement to ban those who make us uncomfortable—and I have been suggesting throughout that *that* is their primary misdeed—can be encapsuled in two institutional expressions: the jail for the involuntary prophet and, more and more, the supermax prison for the intractable voluntary prophet.

We have given attention to the "waste management" function of the local jail, but I would like now to look more closely into the phenomenon of the supermax prison in America, the high security prisons in Great Britain, and other impregnable facilities such as La Santé in Paris that are aimed to house "the worst of the worst."[34]

What are the motivations for this phenomenon? Why isolate in separate, rigidly controlled facilities prisoners already serving lengthy or terminal sentences in secure detention? One clue is revealed in the case of Mumia Abu-Jamal, of whom we spoke earlier, relegated to a supermax prison after the publication of his indictment, *Live from Death Row*. Recall his contention, that "a silent inmate" is preferable to a vocal one. We have also mentioned numerous politically active prisoners, such as Angela Davis, whose agitation for institutional change and whose attempts to communicate with forces bent on control of the marginal precipitated their removal to segregated units reserved for the mentally unstable.

The fact that persons such as Abu-Jamal and Davis are determined and manifestly critical opponents of entrenched racial bias surfaces one of the underlying motivations for the construction of these official dungeons. For the supermax was inaugurated as a response of penal administrators to "the radical civil rights movement of the 1970s."[35] Harlow adds that one of its evident purposes is to utilize political claustration by sequestering "opposition leadership from its base of popular support in the larger community."[36] She expands this to highlight a fact we have witnessed in many of the communiques of formerly apolitical prisoners: they were radicalized by the causes and conditions of their confinement. Phrased differently, penal institutions, already an adjunct of "the state's coercive apparatus of physical detention and ideological containment," often morph into critical repositories "within which, indeed from out of which, alternative social and political practices of counterhegemonic resistance movements are schooled."[37] Thus the need for tomb-like structures in which radical and influential voices for resistance can be muffled in impregnable and inaudible solitude.

To be remanded to such a facility normally means a long-term, indefinite sentence, potentially for the rest of the prisoner's life.[38] Abu-Jamal describes the daily regimen in a supermax:

> A typical day begins at 6:25 a.m. A guard enters a "pod" and announces "yard" ... By 7:05, "yard" is allowed. "Yard" is a euphemism—it actually means "cage," because men go into the cages there ... That ... period lasts for one hour. Then one goes back to his cell, and unless you have a visitor, you don't leave that cell until 7:05 the next morning. It's twenty-three hours lock-in, one hour outside, five days a week. On weekends, it's twenty-four hours lock-in.[39]

Undoubtedly, there are more than political reasons for literally burying a segment of the confined population. The guidelines established by the Federal Bureau of Prisons for the first of these carceral fortresses—in Marion, IL, where the remaining prisoners from the supermax prototype, Alcatraz, were transferred in 1972—state that the goal was behavior modification. It was "designed to assist the individual in changing his attitude and behavior so he may be returned to a regular institutional program."[40]

Some of those in these bunker-like boxes have committed serious acts of violence in a state prison and hence could be considered to need "a change of attitude," but the evidence reveals that it is not specific acts that catalyze officials to "disappear" certain individuals. For example, in the massive supermax at Pelican Bay, California (1,055 cells), in 2010, more than five hundred prisoners had spent at least ten years living in perpetual isolation. Yet not one "of those five hundred was held because of a specific crime committed inside or outside prison." Rather, officials had alleged that all were dangerous gang members "based on their tattoos, books, letters, or drawings."[41] Laurna Rhodes adds her voice to spotlight this clandestine and vengeful practice. The prisons are intended to dissolve "problems" from the main penal population into areas where a "specialized expertise" is the norm. She adds that "supermax placement is rarely determined by the crime for which an inmate is sentenced."[42]

Given this often-surreal function, these "meta prisons" reveal that they are designed to "redouble" the punitive regimen the penitentiary normally inflicts, directed to "those most recalcitrant to it." In this way the "gaps, failings, and contradictions" of the penal culture "can be made to disappear."[43]

The National Institute of Corrections emphasizes that those restrained in these units "have been identified through an administrative rather than a disciplinary process as needing such control on grounds of their … seriously disruptive behavior in other high security facilities."[44] Such foundational statements reveal that, as we have seen in cases as disparate as that of Angela Davis and Joseph Giarratano, a politically disruptive captive can be removed from "normal" detention by administrative fiat since the criteria for transfer allow for wide discretion by administrators. This shields them from the attenuated "due process protection" that must normally be provided a detainee before being placed in punitive segregation.[45]

Kurki and Morris corroborate this "creative" tactic in maintaining that "many supermaxes have been built for political reasons rather than to meet correctional needs."[46] In fact, they note that much of the support for these prisons comes from the ever-vacillating body of opportunistic legislators keen to the equally vacillating play of public opinion and it's fear of super-predators, whether or not there is justification for this label.[47] The authors actually make a case for such prisons "for the incorrigibly violent or unmanageable at the federal level," but there is, in their opinion, not a single one of the state facilities that is justifiable: "all are a grave error in the sad tale of man's brutality to man."[48]

Of course, whether or not those subjected to these inhumane conditions had a diagnosed condition of intellectual disability, the experience of years in total isolation is psychologically devastating. In her analysis of prolonged solitary confinement, Lisa Guenther points to the fracturing of what Husserl calls the "founding stratum of human experience." She notes that the loss of "co-inhabitants of a shared world does not merely change the sign of the world ... it actually erodes the inmate's capacity to perceive objects clearly, and to sustain a coherent, harmonious experience of simple objects."[49]

The inauguration of prisons within prisons to satisfy the anxiety of the powerful to ideas and people who, while in some instances may be seeped in anger and violent tendencies, are, for the most part, projections of inner fears of the prophets whose message cuts too deeply to tolerate. Rhodes thus sees the rise of the supermax not so much as a novelty but as a continuation and extension of a warlike culture that has militarized everything from the schools to the conduct of the police.[50] War imagery and militarism dominate penal culture. In conjunction with the frequently employed "governing through crime" policy that benefits from an inflamed and destructive populist backlash to exert forcible control without addressing structural deficiencies, she contends that the supermax coincides with the merciless aggression often shown to national enemies, both domestic and foreign, who merit such extreme measures "and must be placed beyond the reach of empathy or law."[51]

We conclude our remarks with the reminder that these prisons are the logical extension of the practice of confining those who bedevil us begun with the sixteenth-century workhouse, the seventeenth-century asylum, and the penitentiary of the late eighteenth and nineteenth centuries. Institutions intended to muzzle the prophetic in its many guises have every incentive "to make and remake, label and relabel" a population that fits this spectral category.

Put another way, the supermax is but an exclamation point upon the policy to erect jails and prisons; all of which, then and now, are, to a significant degree, a synonym for the elimination of those whose disconcerting presence and message cannot be tolerated by the fearful, the self-satisfied, and the powerful.

Conclusion

We began our study by asking a question and stating a premise. The question was why so many people classed as intellectually handicapped spend their days, not in therapeutic settings, or in group homes, or under the care of a counselor or therapist, but in jail and prison cells. We then proceeded to state the premise that those so "handicapped," at the least, make those of us in "polite society" uncomfortable, and more commonly, threaten and terrify us. It should now be no secret that our penal facilities are literally overwhelmed by people whose cognitive machinery computes the meaning of their and our lives through a lens crafted by psychological and spiritual perceptions far different than that of the "normal" man or woman.

This leaves us with a paradoxical challenge: either we continue to indulge our alarm and, frankly, disgust at this population and continue to support and underwrite its forced removal from civic participation, or we realize that it is *our* cognitive and ethical structures that require reformation. We must, hearkening back to the moral treatment phenomenon, change our thought patterns to see no ontological, moral, or (for the most part) organic difference between us and them. Furthermore, we must then "think" them out of confinement and imagine them living side by side with us before their enforced exile and debasement can come to an end. The latter presents a daunting challenge on two fronts: for those who have been expelled from the social world and for those who in one way or another underwrite their expulsion.

For the free community, it requires socioeconomic, psychological, therapeutic, and spiritual amendment. As to the first, as Brenner argues, "it is … through the controlling instrument of the economy that the vast majority of social *and* individual objectives are achieved."[1] The economic colossus, especially in the regnant neoliberal philosophy, with its Social Darwinist roots, has laid a crushing burden on the world's poor: the hapless and desperate who both figuratively and literally cling to unstable and deadly rafts in a sea of indifference and, often, hostility as they hope against hope that a better life lies for them somewhere. And it is the objective of the overarching ethos of human worth computed in pounds, or dollars and cents analysis—linked organically to governmental policy—to allow this massive human drift to continue unabated. Part and parcel of its global objective is the destruction of all prophetic voices and movements for organization to redress this sentence of penury and marginality, notably in, but not restricted to, the field of labor.[2]

Economic decisions open the door to virtually limitless profit and opportunity for some and acute social disintegration for countless others. As for the latter, fiscal policy, bolstered by its political allies, has defined this disintegration not in self-critique for the plight of the starving and repressed, but to a large degree in terms of deviant conduct. As we have argued, especially in terms of the voluntary and involuntary prophets whose stories have filled the pages of this book, their criminality is measured, in most cases, not in terms of violent outbursts or willful destruction but on whether they are willing to conform, peacefully and silently, to "the normative ... patterns of behavior that are expected of people playing particular roles in the society."[3] And, as John Lofland insists, the concepts of the deviant and the "crazy" are fixed roles in the civic drama. These stereotypes must exist in the conceptual framework of the personal and collective mind before a set of human beings conforms to the contours of the definition and triggers the adverse response. How else could the current social psychology function without pre-determined categories comparing the "good life" and the "bad life," or the mentally stable and the pathologically unstable?[4]

We have traced the origin of the "criminogenic" personality pattern to the birth of mercantilism and, later, capitalism, with the constituting of workhouses to sweep the English cities and by-ways of "riffraff" incapable of insertion into an economy and ethos based upon profit and useful labor. Then, just as now, this host of poor, mainly unskilled, men and women are forced into confinement not due to their antisocial tendencies but, in many cases, due to their "fantasticall imaginacions," their predilection for the occult, the mysterious, and transrational. Madness, as often as not, is the appellation that has sealed their fate.

These patterns are economically and socially determined but contain a deeper source for their ministration, one that touches upon the second transformation needed regarding the poor, the homeless, and those with an ideational and imagal structure regarded as too extreme to be tolerated publicly. We speak here of a psychic malady among the "sane" that must be confronted and overcome. There is an inherent sadness, loneliness, and alienation from the inner life among the respectable and comfortable that hides behind the mirage that their world is ordered and their elaborate future goals and plans realizable. Emil Brunner speaks of the "naïve human being," made so not for lack of care about his or her life and livelihood but "by the fact that they regard their "knowledge of human existence as settled."[5]

From this viewpoint, the source of existential angst can be assuaged by isolating any people or ideas that would challenge such naivete and insist, in prophetic fashion, that, like Poe's "Masque of the Red Death," the terminal and life usurping plague is inside of ourselves, not them.

Recalling Kierkegaard once again, what the triumphant, autonomous, yet ever wary self lacks "is surely reality." The fabricated illusion of an unreflective, materialist existence is an escape from the dread of obedient submission to forces far greater than any of us, an unwillingness "to submit to the necessary in oneself, to what may be called one's limit."[6] Although Kierkegaard was deeply opposed to Hegel's philosophy of Spirit and history, they find common ground naming and castigating the elaborate structures of fantasy we create to hide from the overarching presence of the divine, the divine will, and the inescapable transience in which our lives are steeped. Hegel submits that the sciences and seekers of technical knowledge pursue the meaning of phenomena within a pragmatic agenda that seeks the worth "for this specific thing" rather seeking "the ground that answers for everything."[7] They "have never enlarged their hearts (beyond the bustle of finite life) or looked into the pure aether of the soul." Sounding much like Kierkegaard, he then insists that religion is not serene; it "takes its start from anguish, [and] awakens this anguish."[8]

In the same manner, Sartre, too, found the inauthentic life as a "flight before anguish," "an effort at distraction before the future." It maintains an apprehensive dismissal of the reality and consequences of the freedom in which our lives are grounded: "there exists a specific consciousness of freedom; and we wished to show that this consciousness is anguish." If one could openly face the existential abyss, she, like the madman or woman, would need to apprehend herself "as a consciousness which possesses a pre-ontological comprehension of its essence and a pre-judicative sense of its possibilities."[9]

These thoughts suggest the third area of transformation necessary for us to think those with exceptional cognitive and imaginative frameworks out of jail and into a fruitful and caring relationship with the rest of us. It concerns the psychiatric and psychological experts with almost total determinative power to label people as mentally deficient and, all too often, delinquent. This ethos needs to be reframed, first, in terms of appreciating that there are different neurological networks that bring meaning and fulfillment than the one prescinding from the prevailing biological paradigm. A nomos is a foundational lens for apprehending the world that produces normative commitments fully coherent within the scope of the perceiver's consciousness. But how can therapeutic professionals, so ideologically convinced that the methods employed in practicing their craft are right, discover the humility necessary to understand the other?

Fully human encounters are impossible in an "I–it" relation wherein the patient is judged prior to being known. Lacan speaks of this as a negation of the "Word." He argues that psychoanalysis has "only a single intermediary: the patient's word … And every word calls for a reply." He is not speaking of grammar or matter of fact statements but the truth that resides in the heart of the client that must be carefully summoned and appreciated as sacred. Whatever the "symptom" the one under analysis is portraying, "the symptom itself is structured like a language, because the symptom is a language from which the Word must be liberated."[10]

Without an "I–Thou" basis of human interaction, all the defensive mechanisms of the unstable self easily turn into accusations that seek to dispel any intimations of error on the part of the analyst. Luhrmann notes the cut and dry education so many psychiatrists receive, a process of "memorizing the criteria and learning to prototype the categories." In this way, they "learn to talk and act as if the disorders are there in the world, that they are instantly recognizable."[11] It easily leads one to ward off any doubts about the competence of this process. My sanity, in such an interchange, can, in effect, only be solidified in comparison to your lack of the same. As one "madman" proclaims:

> Perfectly aware, as you see, I continued walking along the high road of madness, which was, in fact, the road of my reality, as it now opened before me … But I was crazy because I had, in fact, this precise mirroring awareness of you who also walk along this same street without choosing to be aware of it, you are sane, and the more sane you are, the louder you shout at the one walking beside you: "I, this? I, thus? You're blind! You're crazy."[12]

Jaspers proclaims, however, hearkening back to Lofland, that it is indeed possible "to partake in the inner life of another person through a tentative exchange of roles." Through this imaginative and empathetic construct, by means of "a certain dramatic play," one comes closer to the real that is so easy to avoid in the confident assertions of supposed experts. In Jaspers' mind, this openness enables one to touch something profound within ourselves as well as in the patient.[13] For Foucault, this approach is "therapeutics *par excellence*." For a personalist approach "cures insofar as it is a disregard of all cures." If the patient truly needs to be "cured"—and some pathological states are surely in need of such—if she can be appreciated for who she is, she resumes her place "in the activity of natural beings" and, in that relational equity, "succeeds in being cured."[14] Brunner adds from a theological perspective that "the soul itself … is that which knows" and in "the very act of laying something upon the dissecting table for examination, the soul looks away beyond it."[15]

This insight is reminiscent of the contemporary interpersonal psychology forwarded by Miller and Rollnick. The traditional premise used in the helping professions is that any demonstrative change in the counselee is the result of treatment. The authors contend, by contrast, that it is a growing conviction among many that "positive change often occurs without formal treatment." It occurs, as Foucault suggests, "naturally." Moreover, the process of psychological change can be sped up or facilitated by brief interventions in a more genuine and respectful environment: "The fascinating point is that so much change occurs after so little counseling."[16]

We have spent enough time critiquing the "sanity" associated with common sense and conventional social compromises to retrace our thoughts on how insight can only flourish when ideas that cause an epistemological and moral crisis are given due consideration. Suffice to say that all of this reinforces our conviction that the tragedy of our treatment of the mentally ill can only be addressed substantively by allowing ourselves to see the massive deficiencies in the ever-elastic definition of precisely who is sane and insane and what, precisely, constitutes sanity. The latter would include, reminiscing on Kierkegaard and Merton, facing life and its ominous fragility with equanimity, compassion, and faith. Another approach would be to contemplate Pascal's famous aphorism: "Men are so necessarily mad, that not to be mad would amount to another form of madness."[17]

The fourth area that must be expanded to better understand, respect, and liberate the hundreds of thousands locked away in captivity for failing to act as we expect "sane" people to act is in the area of spirituality. Human beings possess a soul as well as a body and a mind. Even if you are not a believer, the history of psychotherapy up until the time of its demotion before a medicalized psychiatry was established on the primacy of internal impulses, myths, and archetypal symbols that are outside the realm of the physical and temporal. We will use Brunner here, but we have referenced a wide body of sources testifying to the realm of the unconscious and the psychical as "the origin of all genius." Here "in the fiery centre all is still fluid ... Here the truth has not yet been solidified into sharp masculine interpretations, but everything is still maternally soft, in symbols, intuitions, and emotional awareness." This perennial and ontological foundation produces a seeing, an awareness, a feeling that is "close to the primal reality, to that existence and life which has no contradictions, which has not yet been differentiated."[18]

We are speaking here, of course, of the domain where prophecy finds its home—whether voluntary or involuntary. It is expansive in its scope and, although driven by an ideological dualism in its critique of the status quo, its ground is the unity of all things, the sacredness of all things, the divine presence in all things, an irresistible force of love and compassion that will not cease to emit its groans and searing invective until all are treated with the fundamental dignity that is their birthright.

Needless to say, as we have already surfaced, there are many in the world of religion who would strenuously reject to what may appear to them as crypto pantheism. This is not, however, that of which we speak. Rather, we elevate a panentheism; the natural world is not God, but God is at the center of everything. Employing Christian theology, in Christ "all things hold together" (Col. 1:17) and "Christ is all in all" (Col. 3:11).

Kierkegaard calls such faith a miracle but one from which no one is excluded. In it, one can apprehend the truths of reality by means of a relation with the Absolute.[19] The lowly believer is thus the one least susceptible to succumb to the myopia of "optical illusion." For that person "sees with the eyes of faith." He is content "with being himself." Indeed, by not losing himself in the evanescent fantasy of material stability, even though many observers dismiss him as "a lowly person," he does not fully adopt this label. Rather, "by holding fast to God with the reservedness of eternity, he has become himself."[20]

The challenge of faith is by no means an easy one. As Becker points out, the average person finds it dauting to take "the lonely leap of faith." If one has joined self-image to a rigidly materialist or pragmatic worldview, that act of determination and submission becomes a cause of disillusionment.[21] Moreover, faith takes one into a dimension where the entire cognitive machinery derives its impetus from a source outside the realm of the conventional and matter of fact. In its staring point of complete remission of "methodical and systematic" thinking, "religious experience becomes less unusual as it becomes functionally more influential on the conduct of everyday life."[22]

Having spelled out the challenges necessary for a liberation of the prophets and their wounded counterparts from penal control, let us look briefly at what obstacles they will face if we are able to welcome them home.

Even under the best circumstances, prophets must remain faithful to their "nomos," to the understanding of their lives and our lives even if that conclusion does not result in them being carted away in handcuffs. There is a regular temptation, given the difficulty of their lives, "to melt into the collective."[23] Yet, as revealed in Chapter 5, the prophet cannot exist comfortably with the world, whatever its present configuration. Structure, with its requirement of conformity to power relations, as Turner insists, is inevitable at every stage of the growth process. Those of us who are university professors witness an example each year as Seniors prepare to graduate. Many have spent four years under academic pressures, longing for freedom and self-expression. Yet, for all the romantic fantasies of "taking a year off" and traveling or indulging in creative pursuits, the prospect of not immediately getting a job or starting a career is nearly traumatizing. A significant part of this is, of course, economic, but there is a deeper fear of "liminal" space, of exiting the meritocracy for at least a little while. The point here is that the prophet can only exist in liminal space, in what Turner calls "anti-structure."

We have described the intense loneliness and helplessness that define a prophet's life—a solitude she shares with the mystic. She can never be fully at home in her society, and, worse, cannot help furthering her isolation due to her fidelity to the Word. For the latter chafes at the incessant human hunger for comfort and stability, and, regularly, the willingness to ignore, or even cause, suffering upon those whose existence brings doubt upon those captivating pursuits.

For the prophet to find a home, even at the edge of the inside, she must be free to speak and live her truth; and we must, finally, see the illusion in trying to create an environment without a degree of necessary flux and commotion, where discomforting ideas and people are repressed and punished. After all, the prophet is here to save us and to save the world.

The prophet as world saver

The human community in which we live is preternaturally unstable. There are simply too many ideological starting points and systems of belief to allow for uniformity at the macro level. To add to the turmoil, all persons, at least since Descartes and the birth of rationalism, tend to regard themselves as the centre of the world in which they reside. Brunner adds that even where "in theory" one thinks that he or she "has overcome this 'naive anthropocentricism'," in practice, "in life itself," he or she does not cease to assert themselves "as this centre." And from this perspective, there are as many centres as there are human beings resulting in "all the chaos and disintegration in the world."[24]

The human ego, untransformed by inner forces that seek to subdue it, will resort to violence to ward off threats to its imperial designs. This is compounded exponentially by group ego. In his famous monograph, Reinhold Niebuhr argued that specific persons are capable of virtue, even selflessness, but neither are capable at the collective level.[25] We are barbarous as members of groups; the larger they are, the more we feed, economically and politically, on the blood of our victims.

Prophets are the only answer to this carnage. In the secret domain of their hearts, they remind us, first, that the only peace this world can give—both to us as individuals and to us as members of communal associations—will come when we decenter ourselves and place God, or a synonym for the ultimate that drives us to our knees, at the forefront of consciousness. Second, they give witness that grace, providence, and history reveal that violence, racism, economic and environmental exploitation, and xenophobia eat away at the soul and bring social calamities that will inexorably "sweep us away like a dream" (Ps. 90:5).

Marcia Webb is correct in her contention that the "mentally ill may carry within them the genetic codes to heal the world."[26] She echoes the wisdom of the past uttered by Plato: "[M]y friend, how singularly prophetic is the soul!"[27] Plato knew that the rhythms of the universe are not those fabricated by the engineer and that, even in his day, the madness of prophecy was the only hope for creation. It is "the special gift of heaven, and the source of the chiefest blessings among men."[28] He honored the song of the visionaries for they reminded him of the "song of the swans because they are sacred to Apollo, and have the gift of prophecy."[29]

Nor did Nietzsche lack the appreciation for seers from another world. Only they have the wisdom and charisma, the "rapt vision and delightful illusion" to instill in us respect for "the original Oneness, the ground of Being, ever-suffering and contradictory."[30]

Finally, Foucault, who did not honor Christianity but seems to have honored Christ, unites those regarded as mentally inferior to Christ himself in his mission to inaugurate the reign of God upon the earth. Foucault states that Jesus assumed "the stigmata of fallen nature; from poverty to death." The wounds of humanity are the same as the wounds of the Passion which remind us of "wisdom forgotten, and of madness." In the divine humility, Christ, in the Incarnation, descended and assumed the role of "humanity's foil, its hidden alter-ego, madness ... thereby showing that there was nothing inhuman in man that could not be redeemed and saved."[31]

However one names the divine, the ineffable, the archetypal, it has been the argument of this book that it finds its mouthpiece, its stalwart symbol of hidden divinity and empathy for human suffering in the singular geniuses we call prophets. Some are aware of their "gift" and are piercing in their rhetoric and intrepid fidelity to the truth from which so many try to flee. Others are so constrained by poverty, depression, and neglect that their prophetic formulations are more oblique, but none the less penetrating. For they are the face of the suffering God, of Christ who chose to be homeless, and bore the stinging criticism of being mad and consorting with demons. Yet their message goes out to the ends of the earth (Ps. 19:4).

They are the divine answer to the riddle of humanity's tendency to elevate the few and subjugate the many; its tendency to deny necessity and hide in the shadows of conformity; its fear of faith that everyone and everything is sacred and worth our care and compassion. They will always suffer, but must they suffer due to your and my apathy and disregard? They are blessed in heaven, if not on earth. Jesus surely lauds them:

> Blessed are you when people hate you, and when they exclude you, revile you, and defame you on account of the Son of Man. Rejoice on that day and leap for joy, for surely your reward is great in heaven; for that is what their ancestors did to the prophets. (Lk. 6:22–23)

Notes

Introduction

1   George Orwell, *1984* (New York: Signet, 1959) 313.
2   George Orwell, *1984* (New York: Signet, 1959) 313.
3   For a classic account, see Richard Quinney, *The Social Reality of Crime* (Boston: Little Brown, 1970). For a more contemporary reformulation, see Patricia E. Erickson and Stephen K. Erickson, *Crime, Punishment, and Mental Illness: Law and Behavioral Science in Conflict* (New Brunswick: Rutgers University Press, 2008) Ch. 1.
4   Thomas Szasz, *The Myth of Mental Illness* (New York: Hoeber-Harper, 1961). See also R.D. Laing, *The Politics of Experience* (New York: Pantheon, 1967) and *The Divided Self* (New York: Pantheon, 1969).
5   Mary de Young, *An American History of Mental Illness and Its Treatment* (Jefferson and London: McFarland & Company, 2010) 24.
6   "[We] have taken for granted and presupposed that a large and … an especially important faction of prophetic and redemptory religions have lived not only in an acute but in a permanent state of tension with the world and its orders." Max Weber, "Religious Rejections of the World and Their Direction," in *From Max Weber*, ed. and trans. H.H. Gerth and C. Wright Mills (London and New York: Routledge, 2009) 323–359 at 328; "The Social Psychology of the World's Religions" 267–301 at 285.
7   "Excluding Moses … the prophet as a political figure first appears together with the king … we can think of the two as a double replacement for the charismatic judges." Michael Walzer, *In God's Shadow: Politics in the Hebrew Bible* (New Haven: Yale University Press, 2012) 75. David Reid situates this assembly as "pre-classical" as opposed to the "classical" literary prophets such as Isaiah, Ezekiel, and Jeremiah. See *What Are They Saying about the Prophets?* (New York: Paulist, 1980) 9–10.
8   Weber notes that the basic tension in prophetic history has been that between a priestly or prophetic "officialdom" as opposed to the independent warrant of divine appointment associated with the "virtuoso." "Social Psychology," 288. Claus Westermann writes: "The accusations of the prophets before Amos were mostly directed towards a king; they have to be understood against the background of the historical situation, just as the prophetic tradition afterwards is still a part of the historical tradition. Nathan's accusation against David and Elijah's against Ahab have their respective meanings only in the situation in which a threat to Israel arises from the behavior of the king; and it is against this that the accusation is directed." See "God's Judgment and God's Mercy," in *Old Testament Theology: Flowering and Future*, ed. Ben S. Ollenburger (Winona Lake: Eisenbrauns, 2004) 203–221 at 213. Walzer states: "Court and temple prophets speak with the authority of the court and temple which reinforces and, we are likely to think constrains the divine calling." *In God's Shadow*, 87.
9   Walzer, *In God's Shadow*, 87.
10 Cathleen Kaveny, *Prophecy Without Contempt: Religious Discourses in the Public Square* (Cambridge, MA: Harvard University Press, 2016).

11   Ibid. Chs. 4–5. This is not to infer, however, that critical voices raised on behalf of America's vulnerable are always tethered to a nationalist agenda. There are numerous men and women whose motivation and fervent interventions fully align with the understanding of prophecy presented in this book. Kaveny gives many of them credit in the areas of race, pacifism, disarmament, and opposition to torture. That said, I am working with a narrower definition of the prophetic than she presents in her volume.

12   In a classic work, Leon Festinger and his coauthors examine the phenomenon of apocalyptic sects and the cognitive dissonance that often ensues in adherents despite the failure of their prediction of cosmic doom. See Leon Festinger, Henry W. Riecken, and Stanley Schachter, *When Prophecy Fails* (Minneapolis: University of Minnesota Press, 1956).

13   Karl Jaspers, *General Psychopathology*, trans. J. Hoenig and Marian W. Hamilton (Chicago: University of Chicago Press, 1963) 108.

14   George Graham, "Self-Ascription: Thought Insertion," in *The Philosophy of Psychiatry*, ed. Jennifer Raddon (New York: Oxford University Press, 2004) 89–103 at 90.

15   Abraham Heschel, *The Prophets* (New York: Harper & Row, 1955) 204–205.

16   Andrew Scull, *Madhouse: A Tale of Megalomania and Modern Medicine* (New Haven and London: Yale University Press, 2005) 13.

17   Ibid.

18   Henri Bergson, *The Two Sources of Morality and Religion*, trans. Ashley Audra and Cloudesley Brereton (Garden City: Doubleday, 1935) 32.

19   Rudolf Otto, *The Idea of the Holy*, trans. John W. Harvey (New York: Oxford University Press, 1958) 12.

20   Amanda Pustilnik, "Prisons of the Mind: Social Value and Economic Inefficiency in the Criminal Justice Response to Mental Illness," *The Journal of Criminal Law and Criminology* 96 (2005) 217–266 at 265.

21   Loic Wacquant, "Class, Race, and Hyperincarceration in Revanchist America," *Daedalus* 139 (2010) 74–90.

22   "In 1992, the National Alliance for the Mentally Ill (NAMI) and the Public Citizen's Health Research Group released a report that described alarmingly high numbers of people with schizophrenia, bipolar disorder, and other severe mental illnesses incarcerated in jails across the country. The report documented that most of the mentally ill arrested had not committed major crimes but rather misdemeanors or minor felonies directly related to the symptoms of their untreated illnesses." See Erickson et al, *Crime, Punishment, and Mental Illness*, 4.

23   Alex Vitale, *The End of Policing* (London and New York: Verso, 2017) 84.

24   Rene Girard, "Mimesis and Violence," in *The Girard Reader*, ed. James G. Williams (New York: Crossroad, 1996) 9–19.

25   Louis Sass, *Madness and Modernism* (New York: Basic Books, 1992) 1.

26   Leo Strauss, *Early Writings*, trans. Michael Zank (Albany: State University of New York Press, 2002) 76.

Chapter 1

1   Nancy Wolff has studied the rise of mental health courts. Since their inception in 1997, some 300 are now operational in the US. Basing themselves on a "more relationally-sensitive or procedurally-just approach," the therapeutic jurisprudence offered is deemed preferable to subjecting those presumed to be mentally ill to the frequently traumatic dynamics of a criminal trial. However, she found evidence of "a two-track, separate and unequal system of criminal processing where one group of offenders receives authoritative, punitive criminal processing and the other group receives relational, rehabilitative criminal processing." Race and class factors play a significant role in the composition of the relative

groups. She notes a study that reviewed 20 mental health courts "and only four had study samples representative of the general jail population. By contrast, the preponderance of mental health court research analyzed samples that were disproportionately White males in their mid-thirties." See "Are Mental Health Courts Target Efficient?" *International Journal of Law and Psychiatry* 57 (2018) 67–76 at 72.

2 Ministry of Justice, *Costs Per Place and Costs Per Prisoner by Individual Prison* (London: Ministry of Justice, 2019).

3 Christian Henrichson and Ruth Delany, *The Price of Prisons: What Incarceration Costs Taxpayers* (New York: Vera Institute of Justice, 2012) 8.

4 Richard G. Frank and Thomas G. McGuire, "Mental Health Treatment and Criminal Justice Outcomes," in *Controlling Crime: Strategies and Outcomes*, ed. Philip J. Cook, Jens Ludwig, and Justin McCrary (Chicago: University of Chicago Press, 2011) 167–212 at 167. Alisa Roth cites an exchange with the New York City Department of Corrections in which it was communicated to her that in 2010, 30 percent of the detainees on Rikers Island were diagnosed as mentally ill; that number rose to 40 percent in 2014 and 43 percent in 2017. See *Insane: America's Criminal Treatment of Mental Illness* (New York: Basic Books, 2018) 3.

5 Rich Calder, "NYC Jails Spending Rises Despite Population Decline," *New York Post*, January 22, 2019.

6 The Vera Institute of Justice found that incarcerating the mentally ill costs two to three times what community-based treatment does. Sees Alex Vitale, *The End of Policing* (London and New York: Verso, 2017) 76.

7 "The mostly commonly used estimate, that 90% of prisoners have mental health issues, is now 20 years old. The Institute of Psychiatry told us that it estimated that over half of prisoners have common mental disorders, including depression, post-traumatic stress disorder and anxiety. It similarly estimated that around 15% of prisoners have specialist mental health needs." House of Commons Committee on Public Accounts, *Mental Health in Prisons* (House of Commons, 13 December, 2017) 9.

8 Doris J. James and Lauren E. Glaze, *Mental Health Problems of Prison and Jail Inmates* (Washington, DC: Bureau of Justice Statistics, 2006) 1–11 at 1. Roth's research corroborates the government report. See *Insane*, 3. Wolff writes that a meta-analysis of 62 psychiatric surveys reveals that 14 percent of those under correctional supervision, or approximately one million people, have a major mental illness. This does not necessarily contradict the data offered by James and Glaze as well as by Roth but suggests that there are varying interpretations regarding the exact number of the "mentally unstable" in the penal system. See "Are Mental Health Courts Target Efficient?" 70.

9 Pustilnik, "Prisons of the Mind," 218.

10 Ibid. 219. We will look more in detail in Chapter 3 at the circumstances that allow wide discretion in the response of law enforcement to individuals whose comportment prompts complaints from the citizenry. Furthermore, as has been noted, the lack of space in shelters and public institutions leaves jail as a default housing option for those in certain states presumed to be a public nuisance. David Garland adds an explanatory affirmation of this trend: "Large-scale incarceration functions as a mode of economic and social displacement, a zoning mechanism that segregates those populations rejected by the depleting institutions of family, work and welfare and places them behind the scenes of social life. In the same way, for shorter terms, prisons and jails are increasingly being used as a … repository for the mentally ill, drug addicts, and poor, sick people for whom the depleted social services no longer provide adequate accommodation." See *The Culture of Control* (Chicago: University of Chicago Press, 2002) 178–179.

[11] Barbara Taylor, "The Demise of the Asylum in Late Twentieth Century Britain," *Transactions of the Royal Historical Society* 21 (2011) 193–215 at 195.

[12] Shane Levesque, "Closing the Door: Mental Illness, Criminal Justice, and the Need for a Uniform Mental Health Policy," *Nova* 34 (2010) 711–738 at 717.

[13] Craig Haney corroborates this catastrophic trend regarding the mentally suspect: "Because persons with special psychiatric needs now are less likely to be adequately protected by social welfare agencies and other institutions, or to be buffered from the social and economic hardships to which their disabilities make them vulnerable, their numbers in the criminal justice system have grown. Thus, the criminal justice system has filled the void left by the drastic reductions in public mental health programs." See *Reforming Punishment* (Washington, DC: American Psychological Association, 2006) 244–245.

[14] Pustilnik suggests the 12-month number. See "Prisons of the Mind," 234, while James and Glaze put the number at five months. See *Mental Health Problems of Prison and Jail Inmates*, 8.

[15] Levesque, for one, writes of the "trauma" to which the incarcerated "insane" are repeatedly subjected and the inaccessibility of adequate social and psychological services. The effect, he claims, exacerbates, or even creates, mental instability. See "Closing the Door," 723.

[16] Max Weber notes that prophets were summoned mainly by acoustic as opposed to visual experiences. They were charged "with a mission to communicate, possibly also to perform." See *Ancient Judaism* (London: George Allen and Unwin, 1952) 312.

[17] Daniel Robinson, *Wild Beasts and Idle Humors: The Insanity Defense from Antiquity to the Present* (Cambridge, MA and London: Harvard University Press, 1996) 8. In the "Ion," Socrates tells Ion, who argues for Homer's excellence above all poets in revealing things hidden: "the gift which you possess of speaking excellently of Homer is not an art, but … an inspiration; there is a divinity moving you." See Plato, "Ion" in *Dialogues of Plato*, Vol. I, trans. Benjamin Jowett (New York: Oxford University Press, 1892) 497–511 at 501.

[18] Plato, "Ion," 502. Weber writes that the prophet "was nothing but a means of communication of divine imperatives. He always remained a tool and servant of his respective mission." See *Ancient Judaism*, 299.

[19] Robinson, *Wild Beasts and Idle Humors*, 76.

[20] Joel Gold and Ian Gold, *Suspicious Minds: How Culture Shapes Madness* (New York: Free Press, 2014) 17.

[21] Martha Nussbaum, *The Fragility of Goodness* (Cambridge: Cambridge University Press, 1986) 201.

[22] Plato, "Phaedrus," in *Six Great Dialogues*, trans. Benjamin Jowett (Mineola: Dover, 2007) 93–139 at 108.

[23] Roy Porter, *Madmen: A Social History of Madhouses, Mad Doctors and Lunatics* (Stroud: Tempus, 2004) 30–31.

[24] Desiderius Erasmus, *The Praise of Folly* (New York: Walter J. Black, 1942) 240.

[25] "Poor vagabonds, criminals, and 'deranged minds' would take the part played by the leper." Michel Foucault, *Madness and Civilization*, trans. Richard Howard (New York: Vintage, 1973) 7.

[26] Stephen A. Diamond, *Anger, Madness, and the Daimonic: The Psychological Genesis of Violence, Evil, and Creativity* (Albany: State University Press of New York, 1996).

[27] Porter, *Madmen*, 20–21; Foucault, *Madness*, 62.

[28] Foucault, *Madness*, 82.

[29] Porter, *Madmen*, 279.

[30] Foucault, *Madness*, 8–9.

[31] Peter Sedgwick, *Psycho Politics* (New York: Harper & Row, 1982) 135; Andrew Scull, *Social Disorder/Mental Disorder* (Berkeley: University of California Press, 1989) 17.

[32] I am reminded here of the work of Rowan Williams. He writes that drawing "up a 'map' illustrating the dependent or contingent character of all we experience leaves a question not about how we provide an extra piece of causal explanation but about whether this style of description needs a context or frame that cannot be categorized within the limits of the discourse we have been using." See *The Edge of Words* (London and New York: Routledge, 2014), 18.

[33] Foucault, *Madness*, 6.

[34] There was a cadre of saints (St. Foy, St. Leonard, St. Quentin, Mary Magdalene, Our Lady of Rocamadour) whose sole heavenly task was to free prisoners, whether justly incarcerated or not. The simple fact of human neglect and suffering was enough to stir divine compassion and charge the saints with a liberating mission. The high Middle Ages saw not only these direct interventions but also, as a result, numerous towns in Europe would free condemned prisoners on the specific town's saint's day. Jean Dunbabin writes: "Here there was a clear assertion that humans could rightly judge where mercy should be shown; but it was set in the broader context of a religious gesture that firmly put divine love above human law, at least for one day." See *Captivity and Imprisonment in Medieval Europe* (Houndmills: Palgrave Macmillan, 2002) 138–139. James Whitman reminds us that the medieval ordeal, for all of its pathos and near comedic formality, was not about discovering evidence but freeing humans from the "fearsome" moral consequences of testifying and thus bringing harm upon another, even if it was patently obvious that the offender was culpable. See *The Origins of Reasonable Doubt* (New Haven: Yale University Press, 2000) 211–212.

[35] C.G. Jung, "The Collective Unconscious," in *The Collected Work of C.G. Jung*, Vol. 9, trans. R.F.C. Hull (Princeton: Princeton University Press, 1968) I, 87–99.

[36] Commenting upon Weber's thesis regarding Protestantism and the apotheosis of capitalism as the new civil religion, Eugene McCarraher writes: "The 'elective affinities' of Protestantism and capitalism originated in the repudiation of Catholic sacramentalism—a Christianized form, [Weber] implied, of the earlier enchanted universe, a cultic ensemble of rituals and relics in which matter and human relationships were believed capable of mediating the supernatural." See *The Enchantments of Mammon: How Capitalism Became the Religion of Modernity* (Cambridge, MA: The Belknap Press of Harvard University Press, 2019) 7.

[37] Austin Van der Slice, "Elizabethan Houses of Correction," *Journal of Criminal Law and Criminology* 45 (1936) 45–67 at 47.

[38] Ibid. 48; Michael Ignatieff, *A Just Measure of Pain* (New York: Pantheon, 1978) 11–12.

[39] Zygmunt Bauman comments on this decisive historical shift in his observation of the transition from the community based social control that governed the early Middle Ages to the "absolutist state" whose roots were firmly planted in the adverse reaction to the vast numbers of released feudal laborers that led to the confinement of vagabonds and "masterless men." See "Legislators and Interpreters," in *Intimations of Postmodernity* (London: Routledge, 1991) 1–25 at 5–6.

[40] Ibid. 51–52. See also Randall McGowen, "The Well-Ordered Prison," in *The Oxford History of the Prison*, ed. Norval Morris and David Rothman (New York: Oxford University Press, 1995), 79–109 at 83–84; Thorsten Sellin, *Slavery and the Penal System* (New York: Elsevier, 1976) 71–74.

[41] Van der Slice, "Elizabethan Houses," 54.

[42] Ibid. 53; Ignatieff, *A Just Measure*, 31–37; Sellin, *Slavery and the Penal System*, 73.

[43] Van der Slice, "Elizabethan Houses," 54. For a comparison of the functions of the jail and workhouse, see Ignatieff, *A Just Measure*, 30–34. See also Jennifer Graber, *The Furnace of Affliction* (Chapel Hill: University of North Carolina Press, 2011) 17–18.

44 John Irwin, *Jail* (Berkeley: University of California Press, 1986) Ch. 1.

45 Quoted in Ignatieff, *A Just Measure*, 25.

46 "Peasants have always been inclined to magic. Their whole economic existence has been specifically bound to nature and has made them dependent on elemental forces. They readily believe in a compelling sorcery directed against spirits who rule over or through elemental forces." Weber, "Social Psychology," 283.

47 Van der Slice, "Elizabethan Houses," 45–46.

48 Scull, *Social Disorder*, 218.

49 Quoted in Ignatieff, *A Just Measure*, 26.

50 Thomas Freeman, "The Rise of Prison Literature," *Huntington Library Quarterly* 72 (2009) 133–146 at 137–138.

51 Bauman, "Legislators and Interpreters," 6–9.

52 Scull, *Social Disorder*, 219.

53 Foucault, *Madness*, 46.

54 Ibid. 186.

55 Ibid. 186.

56 Scull, *Social Disorder*, 216.

57 John Lofland, *Deviance and Identity* (Englewood Cliffs: Prentice Hall, 1969) 14.

58 John Witte, *God's Joust, God's Justice: Law and Religion in the Western Tradition* (Grand Rapids: Eerdmans, 2006) 289–291.

59 Foucault, *Madness*, 57.

60 Ibid. 205.

61 Jaspers, *General Psychopathology*, 1.

62 P.H. Pinel, *A Treatise on Insanity*, trans. D.D. Davis (New York: Hafner, 1962) 4 [orig. pub. 1806].

63 Pinel writes that "coercion must always appear to be the result of necessity, reluctantly resorted to and commensurate with the violence or petulance it is intended to correct." Ibid. 67–68.

64 Ibid. 67.

65 Ibid. 5.

66 Samuel Tuke, *Description of the Retreat* (London: Dawsons of Pall Mall, 1964) vi [orig. pub. 1813].

67 Ibid. 134.

68 Ibid. 149.

69 Scull, *Social Disorder*, 98–99.

70 Quoted in Heather Vacek, *Madness: American Protestant Responses to Mental Illness* (Waco: Baylor University Press, 2015) 75.

71 Ibid.

72 Quoted in ibid. 72–73.

73 Scull, *Social Disorder*, 105–106.

74 David Rothman, *The Discovery of the Asylum* (Boston: Little Brown, 1971) 126.

75 Connolly supervised the Hanwell Asylum in Middlesex beginning in the 1840s. He wrote of the compassionate tenor of the institution stating that "wherever [inmates] go, they meet kind people and hear kind words; they are never passed without some recognition, and the face of every officer is the face of a friend." Taylor, "The Demise of the Asylum," 202.

76 Robert Whitaker, *Mad in America: Bad Science, Bad Medicine, and the Enduring Mistreatment of the Mentally Ill* (Cambridge, MA: Perseus, 2002) 29.

77 Gold and Gold, *Suspicious Minds*, 25.

78 Scull, *Social Disorder*, 308.

[79] Vacek, *Madness*, 86.

[80] Scull, *Social Disorder*, 16.

[81] Rothman, *The Discovery of the Asylum*, 151.

[82] Gold and Gold, *Suspicious Minds*, 25.

[83] Ibid.

[84] Porter, *Madmen*, 195.

[85] John Locke, *An Essay Concerning Human Understanding* (Oxford: Clarendon, 1924) II, I, 2.

[86] Vacek, *Madness*, Ch. 2; Ignatieff, *A Just Measure*, 70–71.

[87] Porter, *Madmen*, 45.

[88] Gold and Gold, *Suspicious Minds*, 31; Anne Harrington, *Mind Fixers: Psychology's Troubled Search for the Biology of Mental Illness* (New York: W.W. Norton, 2019) 3.

[89] Gold and Gold, *Suspicious* Minds, 32; John M. Neale and Thomas F. Oltmanns, *Schizophrenia* (New York: John Wiley & Sons, 1980) 3.

[90] Neale and Oltmanns, *Schizophrenia*, 4–5.

[91] Jason Schnittiker, Michael Missoglia, and Christopher Uggan, "Out and Down: Incarceration and Psychic Disorders," *Journal of Health and Social Behavior* 53 (2012) 448–464 at 450: Michal Gottfredson and Travis Hirschi, *A General Theory of Crime* (Palo Alto: Stanford University Press, 1990). Bonita Veysey and her coauthors make a similar argument: "What we call schizophrenia is often the result of a certain kind of childhood development with respect to rule-following. Normally, the child leans his basic repertory of rules through loving submission to adult authority … If the adult is uncaring, or is not respected by the child, we witness the development of the coercive megalomania so typical of the … schizophrenic … Not having a rule-maker he can respect, the young person becomes his own lawgiver." Bonita M. Veysey, Johanna Christian, and Damian J. Martinez, "Identity Transformation and Offender Change," in *How Offenders Transform Their Lives*, ed. Bonita M. Veysey, Johanna Christian, and Damian J. Martinez (Cullompton: Willan, 2009) 114.

[92] Terrie E. Moffit, "Adolescence-Limited and Life-Course Persistent Antisocial Behavior: A Developmental Taxonomy," *Psychological Review* 100 (1993) 674–701 at 678, 685.

[93] Ibid. 680. My critique of criminological literature has been stated in other contexts, but, briefly, criminal theorists, nurtured and promoted in an intellectual environment wherein positivism and behaviorism are normative, take for granted the legitimacy of the law, its criminal definitions, and the association of lawlessness with delinquency or, in this case, psychological malfunction. I am not quibbling with the notion that serious antisocial conduct is related to developmental factors in childhood. What I find objectionable is making lawfulness an independent variable from which diagnoses regarding who and who is not worthy of participation in society are based. The overwhelming statistical profile of the typical criminal, including, of course, the one with a "mental problem," is so overdetermined by racial and economic modifiers that I find it, at best, inconclusive to make a "taxonomy" of those persons who will, almost without fail in Moffit's formulation, turn out to be life course persistent criminals and, *a fortiori*, spend a part, or all of, their lives behind bars.

[94] Ian Loader, "Ice Cream and Incarceration: On Appetites for Security and Punishment," *Punishment and Society* 11 (2009) 241–257.

[95] One study of 750 inmates awaiting trial in England and Wales, representing 9.4 percent of all male detainees, discovered that 63 percent suffered from psychological disorder. Of those interviewed, 414 were determined to be in need of immediate treatment even though the authors concluded that the facilities wherein they were held had scant resources to address their diagnosis. See D. Brook, C. Taylor, J, Gunn, and J. Maden,

"Point Prevalence of Mental Disorder in Unconvicted Male Prisoners in England and Wales," *British Medical Journal* 313 (December 14, 1996) 1524–1527.

[96] Jock Young, *The Exclusive Society* (London: Sage, 1999) 54.

[97] Ibid. 154.

[98] Graham, "Self-Ascription/Thought Insertion," 90.

[99] Katherine M. Boydell, Elaine Stasiulis, Brenda M. Gladstone, Tiziana Volpe, Jean Addington, Paula Goehring, et, "Recognition of Psychosis in the Pathway to Mental Health Care," in *Hearing Voices: Qualitative Inquiry in Early Psychosis*, ed. Katherine M. Boydell and H. Bruce Ferguson (Waterloo, Ontario: Wilfred Laurier University Press, 2012) 9–24 at 9.

[100] Eric Kandel, *The Disordered Mind* (New York: Farrar, Strauss, and Giroux, 2018) 85.

[101] Bauman, "Legislators and Interpreters," 15.

[102] Harrington, *Mind Fixers*, 4–5.

[103] Ibid. 32–33.

[104] "Prison and jail officials ... have few options. Although they are neither equipped nor trained to do so, they are required to house hundreds of thousands of seriously mentally ill inmates. In many cases, they are unable to provide them with psychiatric medications. The use of other options, such as solitary confinement or restraining devices, is sometimes necessary and may produce a worsening of symptoms." E. Fuller Tory, Mary T. Sdanovicz, Aaron D. Kinnard, H. Richard Lamb, Donald F. Eslinger, Michael C. Biosotti, and Doris A. Fuller, *The Treatment of Persons with Mental Illness in Prisons and Jails: A State Survey* (Arlington: Treatment Advocacy Center, 2014) 8.

[105] Vitale, *The End of Policing*, 68. Scull writes: "Psychiatric involvement with such unrewarding cases can now be reduced to the occasional prescription of psychoactive drugs to be dispensed by others ... And with the miracles of modern psychopharmacology at hand, our contemporary madhouse keepers possess a restraint with which to subdue their charges, less blatant than the chains and straightjackets employed by their counterparts two centuries ago, and, in consequence, all the more desirable." See *Social Disorder*, 328–329.

[106] Roth, *Insane*, 121.

[107] Ibid. 121–122.

[108] John L. Reed and Maggi Lyne, "Inpatient Care of Mentally Ill People in Prison: Results of a Year's Program of Semi-structured Inspection," *British Medical Journal* 320 (April 15, 2000) 1031–1034 at 1032.

[109] Frank K. Willets and Donald M. Crider, "Religion and Well-Being: Men and Women in the Middle Years," *Review of Religious Research* 29 (1988) 281–294 at 281.

[110] John Swinton, *Spirituality and Mental Health Care: Rediscovering a "Forgotten" Dimension* (London: Jessica Kingsley, 2001) 40–41.

[111] Rodney Stark, Loir Kent, and Daniel P. Doyle, "Religion and Delinquency: The Ecology of a 'Lost' Relationship," *Journal of Research in Crime and Delinquency* 19 (1982) 4–24 at 22.

[112] Philip Rieff, *The Triumph of the Therapeutic* (New York: Harper, 1968) 32.

[113] Sigmund Freud, *The Future of an Illusion*, trans. James Strachey (New York: Norton, 1961); *Civilization and its Discontents*, trans. James Strachey (New York: Norton, 1989). Rieff, *The Triumph of the Therapeutic*, 31.

[114] Sigmund Freud, *Beyond the Pleasure Principle*, trans. C.J.M. Hubback (London: International Psychoanalytic Press, 1922) IV. Max Scheler acknowledged the influence of Freud on his thinking. Here he shows his affirmation of the integrity of instinctual drives: "It is impossible that instincts are the product of sensory experience. The sensory experience only triggers the rhythmically definite sequence of instinctive behavior ... it is impossible to reduce an instinct to the inheritance of characteristics acquired through habit or training." See *Man's Place in Nature*, trans. Hans Meyerhoff (Boston: Beacon, 1961) 18–19.

[115] Freud, *Beyond the Pleasure Principle*, IV.

[116] Ibid. VI.

[117] "In our opinion a presentation which seeks to estimate, not only the topographical and dynamic, but also the economic element is the most complete that we can at present imagine, and deserves to be distinguished by the term meta-psychological." Ibid. I.

[118] Ibid. IV.

[119] Ibid. III.

[120] C.G. Jung, "Concept of the Collective Unconscious," in *The Collected Works of C. G. Jung*, Vol. 9 Part 1, trans. R.F.C. Hull (Princeton: Princeton University Press, 1968) 42–53.

[121] Carl G. Jung, *Man and His Symbols* (New York: Dell, 1968) 78.

[122] Karl Jung, *The Red Book*, trans. Mark Kyburz, John Peck, and Sonu Shandaasani (New York: Norton, 2009) 229.

[123] Jung, *Man and His Symbols*, 88–89.

[124] Ibid. 80.

[125] Anne and Barry Ulanov, *Religion and the Unconscious* (Philadelphia: Westminster, 1975) 219, 225.

[126] Ann Bedford Ulanov and David H. Rosen, *Madness and Creativity* (College Station: Texas A&M Press, 2013) 72.

[127] Rieff, *Triumph of the Therapeutic*, 36.

[128] Jacques Lacan, *Speech and Language in Psychoanalysis*, trans. Anthony Wilden (Baltimore: Johns Hopkins University Press, 1968) 6.

[129] Daniel Senior, "Autobiography of an Incarcerated Sex Offender," December 12, 2016, *American Prison Writing Archive*, www.hamilton.edu/academics/centers/digital-humanities-initiative/projects/american-prison-writing-archive

[130] Erickson et al, *Crime, Punishment, and Mental Illness*, 2.

[131] Harrington, *Mind Fixers*, 126–127.

[132] Gold and Gold, *Suspicious Minds*, 42, 48–49.

[133] Scull, *Social Disorder*, 95.

[134] Harrington, *Mind Fixers*, 97–98.

[135] While often critical of the use of medications for psychiatric patients, Roth notes that procedures such as brain scans have improved the ability to treat symptoms rather than simply sedating troublesome patients. See *Insane*, 11.

[136] Ibid. 102.

[137] T.M. Luhrmann, *Of Two Minds* (New York: Knopf, 2001) 47–48.

[138] Lawrence C. Rubin, "Merchandising Madness: Pills, Promises, and Better Living through Chemistry," *Journal of Popular Culture* 38 (2004) 369–383 at 371–372.

[139] Paula Caplan, *They Say You're Crazy: How the World's Most Powerful Psychiatrists Decide Who's Normal* (Reading, MA: Addison Wesley, 1995) xvii; Rubin, "Merchandising Madness," 371–372.

[140] Emma Frankham, "Victim or Villain: Racial/Ethnic Differences in News Portrayals of Individuals Killed by Police," *Sociological Quarterly* 61 (2020) 231–253.

[141] Grant Gillet, "Brain Pain: Psychic Cognition, Hallucinations, and Delusions," in *The Philosophy of Psychiatry*, 21–35 at 27.

[142] Ladaro Pennix, "4A4L-Uncensored," April 21, 2014, *American Prison Writing Archive*, www.hamilton.edu/academics/centers/digital-humanities-initiative/projects/american-prison-writing-archive

[143] Robert Richter, "Invisible Physics, My Story," January 12, 2016, *American Prison Writing Archive*, www.hamilton.edu/academics/centers/digital-humanities-initiative/projects/american-prison-writing-archive

[144] Quoted in Joshua Dubler and Vincent W. Lloyd, *Break Every Yoke: Religion, Justice, and the Abolition of Prisons* (New York: Oxford University Press, 2020) 173.

[145] Angela Davis, *Angela Davis: An Autobiography* (New York: International Publishers, 1988) 31–32.

[146] Gold and Gold, *Suspicious Minds*, 52.

[147] Ian S. Evison, "Between the Priestly Doctor and the Myth of Mental Illness," in *On Moral Medicine*, ed. M. Therese Lysaught and Joseph J. Kovta, Jr. (Grand Rapids: Eerdmans, 2012) 828–844 at 833.

[148] Roth, *Insane*, 90.

[149] Franz G. Alexander and Sheldon T. Selesnick, *The History of Psychiatry* (New York: Mentor, 1966) 34.

[150] Rubin, "Merchandising Madness," 373.

[151] Whitaker, *Mad in America*, 164.

[152] Raymond Tallis, *Neuromania, Darwinitis, and the Misrepresentation of Mankind* (London and New York: Routledge, 2016).

[153] John Swinton, "Medication of the Soul: Why Medication Needs Stories," *Christian Bioethics* 24 (2018) 302–313 at 305.

[154] Harrington, *Mind Fixers*, 182.

[155] Gold and Gold, *Suspicious Minds*, 53.

[156] Harrington, *Mind Fixers*, 126–127.

[157] De Young, *An American History of Mental Illness*, 9; Caplan, *They Say You're Crazy*.

[158] Louis C. Charland, "Character: Moral Treatment and Personality Disorders," in *The Philosophy of Psychiatry*, 64–77 at 65.

[159] Russell K. Schutt, *Homelessness, Housing, and Mental Illness* (Cambridge, MA: Harvard University Press, 2011) 143.

[160] De Young, *An American History of Mental Illness*, 10.

[161] Alana Siris, Ryan Holliday, and Carol S. North, *The Evolution of the Classification of Psychiatric Disorders* (Basel: MDPI, 2016) 5–6.

[162] Harrington, *Mind Fixers*, 267.

[163] Ibid. 9–10.

[164] Charland, "Character," 64.

[165] Ibid. 70.

[166] Gold and Gold, *Suspicious Minds*, 52.

[167] Siris et al, *The Evolution of the Classification of Psychiatric Disorders*, 6–7.

[168] Charland, "Character," 70.

[169] Ibid. 72.

[170] Willie Williams, "I've Been Incarcerated for Ten Years," October 28, 2019, *American Prison Writing Archive*, www.hamilton.edu/academics/centers/digital-humanities-initiative/projects/american-prison-writing-archive

[171] Caplan, *They Say You're Crazy*, 185–186.

[172] Richard J. McNally, *What is Mental Illness?* (Cambridge, MA: Belknap Press, 2011) 35.

[173] Harrington, *Mind Fixers*, 267.

[174] Ibid.

[175] Kandel, *The Disordered Mind*, 31.

[176] Roy Branson, "The Secularization of American Medicine," in *On Moral Medicine*, ed. M. Therese Lysaught and Joseph J. Kovta, Jr. (Grand Rapids: Eerdmans, 2012) 12–21 at 14.

[177] Scull, *Social Disorder*, 306–307.

[178] Richard J. McNally would be among those who object to the criminalization of mental illness. He writes that "behavioral problems that conflict with social norms, such as criminal

activity, do not indicate a mental disorder. Although some are mentally ill, committing crimes is insufficient to justify a diagnosis of mental illness." See *What is Mental Illness?* 3–4.

[179] Hannah Bertilsdotter Rosqvist, Anna Stenning, and Nick Chown, "Introduction," in *Neurodiversity Studies: A New Critical Paradigm*, ed. Hannah Bertilsdotter Rosqvist, Anna Stenning, and Nick Chown (London and New York: Routledge, 2020) 1–11 at 1.

[180] Sidney Callahan, "A New Synthesis: Alternative Medicine's Response to Mainstream Medicine and Traditional Christianity, in *On Moral Medicine*, ed. M. Therese Lysaught and Joseph J. Kovta, Jr. (Grand Rapids: Eerdmans, 2012) 22–38 at 16.

[181] William F. May, "Afflicting the Afflicted: Total Institutions," in *On Moral Medicine*, ed. M. Therese Lysaught and Joseph J. Kovta, Jr. (Grand Rapids: Eerdmans, 2012) 853–861 at 857.

[182] Jaspers, *General Psychopathology*, 18.

[183] Gold and Gold, *Suspicious Minds*, 232.

Chapter 2

[1] "I entitle *transcendental* all knowledge which is occupied not so much with objects as with the mode of our knowledge of objects in so far as this mode of knowledge is to be possible *a priori*." Immanuel Kant, *Critique of Pure Reason*, trans. Norman Kemp Smith (New York: St. Martin's, 1965) Introduction VII, B 25, A 12 (italics in original).

[2] Suzanne K. Langer, *Philosophy in a New Key* (Cambridge, MA: Harvard University Press, 1942) 4.

[3] "And now if I were to say, 'It is my unshakable conviction that etc.,' this means in the present case too that I have not consciously arrived at the conviction by following a particular line of thought, but that it is anchored in all my *questions and answers*, so anchored that I cannot touch it." Ludwig Wittgenstein, *On Certainty*, trans. Denis Paul and G.E.M. Anscombe (New York and Evanston: J. & J. Harper, 1969) 103.

[4] Alasdair MacIntyre, *Whose Justice, Which Rationality?* (South Bend: University of Notre Dame Press, 1988).

[5] Rosqvist et al, *Neurodiversity Studies*, 1. Andrea Lollini rhetorically asks: "What if we ascertained, with the advancement of neuroscience, that a very large portion of the human population interacts socially … processes information and stimuli, learns, rationalizes, or makes abstractions with a greater variation than previously postulated? … What if, in the end, we discovered that in our current state we lose a considerable human potential—while simultaneously raising the cost of managing those who do not fit what society considers normal patterns of cognition? In other words, are brain attributes one of the cornerstones on which inequality and injustice are built in Western societies?" See "Brain Equality: Legal Implications of Neurodiversity in Comparative Perspective," *Journal of International Law and Politics* 51 (2020) 69–133 at 70.

[6] Luigi Pirandello, "Six Characters in Search of an Author," in *Pirandello Plays*, trans. Eric Bentley (Evanston: Northwestern University Press, 1970) 65–116 at 84.

[7] Hobbes writes that "if a [person] should talk to me of a round quadrangle; or accidents of bread in cheese; or immaterial substances; or of a free subject; a free will; or any free but free from being hindered by opposition; I should not say he were in an error, but that his words were without meaning; that is to say, absurd." See *Leviathan*, ed. C.B. Macpherson (London: Penguin, 1968) I, v. Hume states: "The hypothesis we embrace is plain. It maintains that morality is determined by sentiment. It defines virtue to be *whatever mental action or quality gives to the spectator the pleasing sentiment of approbation*; and vice the contrary." David Hume, "Concerning Moral Sentiments," in *The Essential David*

Hume, ed. Robert Paul Wolff (New York: Mentor, 1969) Appendix I, 238–244 at 244 (italics in original).

8   For Taylor, the view of the self that is disengaged and in rational control was spearheaded by Descartes. It developed in full with Locke and the Enlightenment. Taylor states that "the 'punctual self' ... gains its control through disengagement. [It] is always correlative of an 'objectification' ... Objectifying a given domain involves depriving it of its normative force for us." See Charles Taylor, *Sources of the Self* (Cambridge, MA: Harvard University Press, 1989) 160.

9   Adam Smith writes: "When I endeavour to examine my own conduct, when I endeavour to pass sentence upon it, either to approve or condemn it, it is evident that, in all such cases, I divide myself, as it were into two persons; and that I, the examiner and judge, represent a different character from that other I, the person whose conduct is examined into and judged of. The first is the spectator, whose sentiments with regard to my own conduct I endeavour to enter into, by placing myself in his situation, and by considering how it would appear to me, when seen from that particular point of view. The second is the agent, the person who I properly call myself, and of whose conduct, under the character of a spectator, I was endeavouring to form some opinion." See *The Theory of Moral Sentiments* (New York: Augustus M. Kelley, 1966) III, I. 2 [orig. pub. 1759]. See also John Milbank, *Theology and Social Theory* (Oxford: Blackwell, 1991) 4; Andrew Skonicki, *Conversion and the Rehabilitation of the Penal System* (New York: Oxford University Press, 2019) 23–24.

10   Robert Cover, "Violence and the Word," *Yale Law Journal* 95 (1986) 1601–1639 at 1606–1607.

11   Ibid. 1609.

12   Robert Cover, "Nomos and Narrative," *Harvard Law Review* 97 (1983) 4–68 at 53.

13   Weber, "Religious Rejections of the World," 334.

14   Kant, *Critique of Pure Reason*, I, I, B 34, A.

15   Langer, *Philosophy in a New Key*, 14.

16   Theodor Adorno, *Negative Dialectics*, trans. E.B. Ashton (New York: Seabury, 1972) 53.

17   Ibid. 73.

18   Adorno places the brunt of his critique on Heidegger since the latter rejected the liberal philosophical tradition and, with his emphasis on being itself, seems, on face value, to be immune to the dualist reductionism that dominates subjectivist theories. However, Adorno insists that any attempt at *prima philosophia* is predicated upon the inferiority of other ways of knowing and is itself dualist. Furthermore, his work proceeds from the contention that there is no such thing as "being" in itself: "Being is not simply the totality of all there is ... But what echoes in the word 'Being' ... means entwinement, not something transcendent to entwinement." Adorno would thus be as critical of the argument in this volume as he is of other attempts at a surreptitious metaphysics. Ibid. 138, 106.

19   Friedrich Nietzsche, "The Genealogy of Morals," in *The Birth of Tragedy and The Genealogy of Morals*, trans. Francis Golffing (Garden City: Doubleday, 1956) I, v.

20   Jacob Burckhardt argues that the new anthropology of autonomous individuality was birthed in the Renaissance and epitomized in the writing of Dante. I am elevating the thought of Nietzsche and Foucault for pointing to the overhaul of the use of power, not to undermine individualism, but to make it the servant of those capable of linking personal security and social advancement to mass obedience to those to whom they have made themselves responsible. See Burckhardt, *The Civilization of the Renaissance in Italy*, trans. S.G.C. Middlemore (Oxford: Phaedon, 1945) Part II.

21   Nietzsche, "Genealogy," III, I, I, iii 2; III, ii ii.

22 Ibid. III, ii, ii.

23 Michel Foucault, *The Order of Things* (New York: Pantheon, 1970) 344–345.

24 Ibid. 367. Among Marx's sage essays, he pre-dates the worldview wherein nature becomes one more thing to conquer in the reformulation of worth in terms of control of lesser substances. See "Estranged Labor," in *The Marx Engels Reader*, ed. Robert C. Tucker (New York and London: W.W. Norton, 1978) 66–81.

25 B.F. Skinner, *Beyond Freedom and Dignity* (New York: Alfred A. Knopf, 1972) 74, 113.

26 Ibid. 58, 61.

27 Veysey et al, "Identity Transformation and Offender Change," 2.

28 D.A. Andrews and James Bonta, *The Psychology of Criminal Conduct*, 5th edition (New Providence: LexisNexis, 2010) 79.

29 James, *Varieties of Religious Experience* (New York: Collier, 1960) Lecture I.

30 Martin Buber, *I and Thou* (New York: Scribner, 1958).

31 R.D. Laing, *The Divided Self* (New York: Pantheon, 1969) 17.

32 Ibid. 20–21. T.M. Luhrmann states that modern medicine functions upon the necessary separation of "a person who is ill from the illness." See *Of Two Minds* (New York: Knopf, 2001) 273.

33 Paulo Freire, *Pedagogy of the Oppressed*, trans. Myra Bergman Ramos, 30th anniversary edition (New York: Continuum, 2005) 61.

34 G.W.F. Hegel, *Phenomenology of Spirit*, trans. A.V. Miller (Oxford: Oxford University Press, 1977) 50.

35 Vico, *The First New Science*, trans. Leon Pompa (Cambridge: Cambridge University Press, 2002) II, XII, 137.

36 Ibid. II, XXXVII, 174.

37 It can, of course, be claimed that prophetic utterances are themselves shrouded in dualism. While this is the case in specific instances of "whitewashing" the other, the overall stance of the literary prophets in the Hebrew Bible was one of a critique aiming at repentance, reconciliation, and acknowledgment of the divine intention to provide care for all, especially those outside the spheres of political and religious influence. This is the predominant interpretation that will be forwarded in this volume. Put differently, those who claim divine authority and promote violence without the aim of reconciliation are false prophets.

38 Adorno, *Negative Dialectics*, 21.

39 Langer, *Philosophy in a New Key*, 11–12.

40 Arthur Schopenhauer, *The World as Will and Representation*, trans. E.F.J. Payne (New York: Dover, 1958) I, 7.

41 Alasdair MacIntyre, *After Virtue* (South Bend: University of Notre Dame Press, 1981) 12, 21.

42 Adorno, *Negative Dialectics*, 21.

43 Ibid. 33.

44 Frankham, "Victim or Villain," 241

45 Vitale, *The End of Policing*, 66.

46 Ibid.

47 Frankham, "Victim or Villain," 240.

48 David Leonhardt, "Mental Health as Crime," *New York Times*, September 4, 2020.

49 Vitale, *The End of Policing*, 66; Robert J. Hacker and John J. Horan, "Policing People with Mental Illness: Experimental Evaluation of Online Testing to De-Escalate Mental Health Crises," *Journal of Experimental Criminology* 15 (2019) 551–569 at 552.

50 Hobbes, *Leviathan*, III, xxxii.

51 Walter Wink writes of the "terminally ill" nature of materialism using the same vocabulary. See *Unmasking the Powers* (Philadelphia: Fortress, 1986) 1–2.

52 Kent Nerbern, *Voices in the Stones: Life Lessons from the Native Way* (Novato, CA: New World Library, 2016) 130–132.

53 James, *Varieties*, Lectures XVI and XVII.

54 Ibid. Lecture I.

55 Ibid.

56 Wolfhart Pannenberg, *Anthropology in Theological Perspective*, trans. Matthew J. O'Connell (Philadelphia: Westminster, 1985) 377.

57 Hegel, *Phenomenology of Spirit*, 70.

58 James, *Varieties*, Lecture 1.

59 George Fox, *The Journal of George Fox* (Oakville: Capricorn Books, 1963) 229.

60 Rosqvist et al, *Neurodiversity Studies*, 1.

61 Christopher Paar, Jr., "Essay on Health," February 11, 2019, *American Prison Writing Archive*, www.hamilton.edu/academics/centers/digital-humanities-initiative/projects/american-prison-writing-archive

62 The topics addressed by metaphysics, such as God, freedom, and immortality, are examples of what Immanuel Kant calls the "pure *a-priori*." See *Critique of Pure Reason*, Introduction, II, B 4.

63 Ibid. Introduction, III, B 6, A 3, B 7.

64 Ibid. Introduction, VI, B 21.

65 Harvey Cox, *The Sacred Canopy* (New York: Macmillan, 1965).

66 Jaspers, *General Psychopathology*, 309.

67 Ibid. 10.

68 Ibid. 309.

69 John Swinton, "Restoring the Image: Spirituality, Faith, and Cognitive Disability," *Journal of Religion and Health* 36 (1997) 21–27 at 23

70 St. John of the Cross, "The Ascent of Mount Carmel," in *The Collected Works of St. John of the Cross*, 3rd edition, trans. Kieran Cavanaugh and Otilio Rodriguez (Washington, DC: Carmelite Institute: 1991) Prologue.

71 Ibid. 114–115.

72 Ibid. III, XXI, i.

73 Schopenhauer, *The World as Will and Representation*, II, 17.

74 Ibid. I, 5.

75 Alfred North Whitehead, *Process and Reality* (New York: Free Press, 1978) 3.

76 Ibid. 10.

77 Richard Rohr, "An Opening and Growing Heart," *Center of Action and Contemplation*, July 18, 2017.

78 Richard Rohr, *Everything Belongs* (New York: Crossroads, 2003) 55–59.

79 St. John of the Cross, *Living Flame of Love*, trans. E. Allison Peers (Ligouri: Ligouri Publications, 1991).

80 Julian of Norwich, *Showings, Long Text*, trans. Edmund Collledge and James Walsh (New York: Harper, 1961) Ch. 27.

81 Marcia Webb, *Toward a Theology of Psychological Disorder* (Eugene: Cascade, 2017) 12.

82 Vacek, *Madness*, 164.

83 Ann and Barry Ulanov, *Religion and the Unconscious* (Philadelphia: The Westminster Press, 1975) 25.

84 Don S. Browning, *Religious Thought and the Modern Psychologies* (Philadelphia: Fortress, 1987) 7.

85 Richard Rohr, *A Spring Within Us* (Albuquerque: CAC Publications, 2016) 199.

86 St. Bonaventure, *The Mind's Road to God* (Grand Rapids: Christian Ethereal Library) Chs. 5, 8.

87 Jean Paul Sartre, *Being and Nothingness*, trans. Hazel E. Barnes (New York: Philosophical Library, 1956) Introduction, VI, lxiv. Heidegger takes a similar approach. He states that "an appearance 'of something' does *not* mean showing-itself; it means rather the announcing-itself by something which does not show itself." See Martin Heidegger, *Being and Nothingness*, trans. John Macquarrie and Edward Robinson (New York: Harper & Row, 1962) 52.

88 Emilie Durkheim, *The Elementary Forms of the Religious Life*, trans. Karen Fields (New York: Free Press, 1995) Bk. II, Ch. 7.

89 M. Harvey Brenner, *Mental Illness and the Economy* (Cambridge, MA and London: Harvard University Press, 1973) 23

90 Branson, "The Secularization of American Medicine," 14.

91 Jaspers, *General Psychopathology*, 812.

92 Rieff, *Triumph of the Therapeutic*, 4.

93 John Polkinghorne, a physicist who is also a priest, has undertaken to substantiate the inherent connection between quantum mechanics and religious faith. See *The Quantum World* (Harmondsworth: Penguin, 1986); *Science and Creation* (London: SPCK, 1988).

94 Bernard Lonergan, *Insight* (New York: Philosophical Library, 1970) 44, xx–xxi.

95 Callahan, "A New Synthesis," 25. Anthony O'Hear, writing from the perspective of a scientific atheist, insists that science and religion have common starting points and thus, "it is clear that at a deep level, science cannot be seen to conflict with religion, if each activity is properly conceived. The one looks at the world in an impersonal way ... while the other takes the whole as given and attempts to see it in terms of personal meaningfulness. Indeed, far from being in a state of mutual conflict ... science and religion could even be seen to be part of a mutually sustaining harmony ... science is always going to strive for ultimate explanations and discoveries, which are beyond human powers to verify or falsify." See "Science and Religion," *The British Journal for the Philosophy of Science* 44 (1993) 505–516 at 514–515.

96 Brenner, *Mental Illness and the Economy*, 246.

97 Jaspers, *General Psychopathology*, 328.

98 Thomas Kuhn, *The Structure of Scientific Revolutions* (Chicago: University of Chicago Press, 1962) 5.

99 Anthony Giddens, *Central Problems of Social Theory* (Berkeley: University of California Press, 1970). Arnold Gehlen describes the "natural attitude" as an "a priori" conception of reality that views the world "as caught in a rhythmic, self-sustaining, circular process of motion." See *Man in the Age of Technology*, trans. Patricia Lipscomb (New York: Columbia University Press, 1980) 13. See also Peter Berger and Thomas Luckmann, *The Social Construction of Reality* (New York: Vintage, 1966) 21.

100 Harrington, *Mind Fixers*, 275–276.

101 Browning, *Religious Thought and the Modern Psychologies*, 60.

Chapter 3

1 Richard Hofstadter, *Social Darwinism in American Thought* (New York: G. Braziller, 1959).

2 James G. Crossley, *Jesus in an Age of Neoliberalism* (Sheffield: Equinox, 2012) 26.

3 Michael Hardt and Antonio Negri, *Empire* (Cambridge, MA: Harvard University Press, 2000).

4 Walter Brueggemann, *Tenacious Solidarity*, ed. Davis Hawkins (Minneapolis: Fortress, 1918) 33.

5 McCarraher, *Enchantments of Mammon*, 664.

[6] I refer here to the classic essay on the "new penology" and how the actuarial methods of the insurance industry have transformed not only access to credit, health care, and acceptance into elite schools of higher learning, but also the dynamics of criminal justice using the methodology of risk. See Malcolm Feeley and Jonathan Simon, "The New Penology," *Criminology* 30 (1992) 449–474.

[7] McCarraher, *Enchantments of Mammon*, 16.

[8] Weber, "Social Psychology," 301.

[9] Weber, "Religious Rejections of the World," 331.

[10] Weber, "Social Psychology," 283.

[11] Karl Polanyi, *The Great Transformation* (Boston: Beacon, 1957) 11.

[12] Ibid. 69.

[13] Weber, "Religious Rejections of the World," 333–334.

[14] Michel Foucault, *Discipline and Punish*, trans. Alan Sheridan (New York: Vintage, 1991) 207.

[15] Frankham, "Victim or Villain," 233.

[16] Wacquant, "Class, Race, and Hyperincarceration," 74.

[17] Ibid. 76–77.

[18] Ibid. 22.

[19] Ibid. 74. The Independent Budget Office of New York City reported that in 2012, the population of the jail system was 57 percent Black and 33 percent Hispanic. See *Annual Budget Report, Fiscal Year 2012* (New York: IBO, 2012).

[20] David Garland, *The Culture of Control* (Chicago: University of Chicago Press, 2002) 178.

[21] Pustilnik, "Prisons of the Mind," 225.

[22] Scull, *Social Disorder/Mental Disorder*, 216.

[23] Brenner, *Mental Illness and the Economy*, 230.

[24] Polanyi, *The Great Transformation*, 3.

[25] Herbert Fingarette, *The Meaning of Criminal Insanity* (Berkeley: University of California Press, 1972) 109.

[26] De Young, *Madness*, 26.

[27] Ibid. 12, 14.

[28] Khalil Gibran Muhammad, *The Condemnation of Blackness* (Cambridge, MA: Harvard University Press, 2010) Ch. 1.

[29] Quoted in C. Holzer, B. Shea, J. Swanson, and P. Leaf, "The Increased Risk of Psychiatric Disorders among Persons of Low Socioeconomic Status," *The American Journal of Psychiatry* 6 (1986) 259–271 at 260.

[30] Neale and Oltmanns, *Schizophrenia*, 292.

[31] Whitaker, *Mad in America*, 168.

[32] Jonathan Metzl, *The Protest Psychosis* (Boston: Beacon, 2009); Anne E. Parsons, *From Asylum to Prison* (Chapel Hill: University of North Carolina Press, 2018) 7–8.

[33] Parsons, *From Asylum to Prison*, 1.

[34] Holzer et al, "The Increased Risk of Psychiatric Disorders," 269.

[35] William H. Fisher, Eric Silver, and Nancy Wolff, "Beyond Criminalization: Toward a Criminologically Informed Framework for Mental Health Policy and Services Research," *Administration Policy in Mental Health and Mental Health Services Research* 33 (2006) 544–557 at 546.

[36] Eoin O'Connell, *Reimagining Homelessness* (Bristol: Bristol University Press, 2020) 43–44. On the criminalization of public spaces in the US see Katherine Beckett and Steve Herbert, *Banished* (Oxford and New York: Oxford University Press, 2010). Vitale writes that for those who have mental illnesses or substance abuse problems, or a combination of the two, "their public presence in parks, subways, and sidewalks seem

more menacing … As a result, police are often called to regulate their behavior. In some cases, a stern warning or an order to go elsewhere suffices. In other cases, a ticket may be written for littering, public urination, or other minor infractions. These tickets are rarely paid and usually result in lots of cycling through courts and jails and additional arrests as a rap sheet of minor offenses and unpaid tickets builds up. These tickets do nothing to improve a person's situation and are usually intended to drive people out of certain spaces more than change their behavior." See *The End of Policing*, 78.

37 Vitale, *The End of Policing*, 78–79.

38 Levesque, "Closing the Door," 718–719

39 Ibid.

40 Fisher et al, "Beyond Criminalization," 545–546.

41 Roth, *Insane*, 234.

42 Vitale, *The End of Policing*, 70.

43 Erving Goffman, "The Moral Career of a Mental Patient," in *Asylums* (Garden City: Anchor, 1961) 125–169 at 133–135.

44 Veysey et al, "Identity Transformation and Offender Change," 29.

45 Goffman, "The Moral Career of a Mental Patient", 133–135.

46 Erickson et al, *Crime, Punishment, and Mental Illness*, 19.

47 Levesque, "Closing the Door," 719.

48 Frankham, Victim or Villain," 234.

49 Fingarette, *The Meaning of Criminal Insanity*, 135.

50 Laing, *The Politics of Experience*, 84.

51 Scull, *Social Disorder/Mental Disorder*, 121–122, 123.

52 Lofland, *Deviance and Identity*, 4, 9, 11.

53 St. John of the Cross, "The Ascent of Mount Carmel," 114–115.

54 Vico, *The First New Science*, III, I, 250.

55 Rieff, *Triumph of the Therapeutic*, 72.

56 Alan Watts, *Behold the Spirit* (New York: Pantheon, 1971) xiv.

57 Rodney Stark, *Why God? Examining Religious Phenomena* (Conshohocken: Templeton Press, 2017) 74.

58 Bruce Vawter, *The Conscience of Israel* (New York: Sheed and Ward, 1961) 33.

59 Virgilio Elizondo, *Galilean Journey: The Mexican American Promise* (Maryknoll: Orbis, 2000) 118–119.

60 Szasz, *The Myth of Mental Illness*, 118–119.

61 Ibid. 11.

62 Lacan, *Speech and Language in Psychoanalysis*, 42–43.

63 Webb, *Toward a Theology of Psychological Disorder*, 50.

64 Karl Rahner, *Theological Investigations Vol. XIII, Theological Anthropology, Christology*, trans. David Bourke (New York: Crossroads, 1975) 123.

65 Quoted in Vacek, *Madness*, 112.

66 Thomas Szasz, *The Second Sin* (Garden City: Anchor, 1974) xvii–xviii.

67 Roth, *Insane*, 21–33.

68 Weber, "Religious Rejections of the World," 350.

69 Ibid. 355.

70 Levert Brookshire, "Cell Block Society Cell Block Academia Part One and Two," October 14, 2016, *American Prison Writing Archive*, www.hamilton.edu/academics/centers/digital-humanities-initiative/projects/american-prison-writing-archive

71 John Braithwaite, *Crime, Shame, and Rehabilitation* (Cambridge: Cambridge University Press, 1989) 5–9. See also, Ian Loader and Richard Sparks, *Public Criminology* (London and New York: Routledge, 2011) 78.

[72] In a recent work, I address in detail my critique of retribution, deterrence, and selsective incapacitation. See Andrew Skotnicki, *Conversion and the Rehabilitation of the Penal System: A Theological Rereading of Criminal Justice* (New York: Oxford University Press, 2019) Ch. 2.

[73] Garland, *Culture of Control*, 180. Some of the texts expressive of a retributive response are Andrew Von Hirsch, *Doing Justice* (New York: Hill and Wang, 1976); Ernest Van den Haag, *Punishing Criminals* (New York: Basic Books, 1975; Herbert Morris, "Persons and Punishment," *The Monist* 52 (1968) 475–501. For an overview of the decline of rehabilitation, see Francis A. Allen, *The Decline of the Rehabilitative Ideal* (New Haven: Yale University Press, 1981).

[74] Andrews and Bonta, *Psychology*, 141.

[75] Carl Rogers, *On Becoming a Person: A Therapist's View of Psychotherapy* (Boston: Houghton Mifflin, 1961).

[76] Browning, *Religious Thought and the Modern Psychologies*, 72–73.

[77] Andrews and Bonta, *Psychology*, 7.

[78] James Whitman, *Harsh Justice* (New York: Oxford University Press, 2003) 23.

[79] Andrews and Bonta, *Psychology*, 11.

[80] Ibid. 131.

[81] Garland, *Culture of Control*, 176.

[82] D.A. Andrews, James Bonta, and J. Stephen Wormith, "The Risk-Need-Responsivity Model (RNR): Does Adding the Good Lives Model Contribute to Effective Crime Prevention," *Criminal Justice and Behavior* 38 (2011) 735–755 at 738.

[83] Francis Cullen, "Taking Rehabilitation Seriously: Creativity, Science, and the Challenge of Offender Change," *Punishment and Society* 14 (2012) 94–114 at 104–106.

[84] Devon R. Polashek, "An Appraisal of the Risk-Need-Responsivity (RNR) Model of Offender Rehabilitation and Its Application in Correctional Treatment," *Legal and Criminal Psychology* 17 (2012) 1–17 at 1.

[85] Skinner, *Beyond Freedom and Dignity*, 18, 27.

[86] Andrews and Bonta, *Psychology*, 434, 449.

[87] Ibid. 443, 444–445.

[88] Ibid. 451.

[89] A.E. Bottoms, "An Introduction to the Coming Crisis," in *The Coming Penal Crisis*, ed. A.E. Bottoms and R.H. Preston (Edinburgh: Scottish Academic Press, 1980) 1–24 at 3.

[90] The authors of the Good Lives Model write that "there is a direct relation between goods promotion and risk management in rehabilitative work." They also echo the influence of Rogers in denying any ontological status to human beings as integral moral agents. Instead, they maintain that there is no assumption in their program "that individuals are inherently or naturally good in an ethical sense." See Tony Ward and Shadd Maruna, *Rehabilitation: Beyond the Risk Paradigm* (London and New York: Routledge, 2007) 107, 115. Cullen and his coauthors insist that virtues can and should be inculcated in the penal environment but, once again, assume, in effect, that if, say the mentally ill person is behind bars, he or she must have done something wrong: "[People], including inmates, have an *obligation* to obey the law, not to harm others, and … societal institutions, including the prison, should be organized to facilitate this goal." See Francis T. Cullen, Jody Sundt, and John Wozniak, "The Virtuous Prison: Towards a Restorative Rehabilitation," in *The American Prison: Imagining a Different Future*, ed. Francis T. Cullen, Cheryl Leo Jones, and Mary K. Strohr (Los Angeles: Sage, 2014) 62–84 at 74 (italics in original). For a detailed critique of rehabilitation, see Skotnicki, *Conversion*, Ch. 4.

[91] Gwen Robinson, "Late-Modern Rehabilitation: The Evolution of a Penal Strategy," *Punishment and Society* 10 (2008) 429–445 at 432.

[92] Ibid. 434–435.

93 Feeley and Simon, "The New Penology"; Jennifer M. Ortiz and Hayley Jackie, "The System is not Broken: It is Intentional," *The Prison Journal* 99 (2019) 484–503.

94 Marie Gottschalk, *Caught: The Prison State and the Lockdown of American Politics* (Princeton: Princeton University Press, 2015) 242.

95 Girard, "Mimesis and Violence," 9–19.

96 Rene Girard, *Violence and the Sacred*, trans. Patrick Gregory (Baltimore: Johns Hopkins University Press, 1977) 12.

97 Girard, "Mimesis and Violence," 16–17.

98 Webb, *Toward a Theology of Psychological Disorder*, 135.

99 Dubler and Lloyd, *Break Every Yoke*, 203–204.

100 Rieff, *Triumph of the Therapeutic*, 40.

101 Rene Descartes, *Meditations on First Philosophy*, trans. Donald Cress (Indianapolis: Hackett, 1993) Meditation 3, 21–27.

102 Soren Kierkegaard, "The Sickness Unto Death," in *Fear and Trembling and The Sickness Unto Death*, trans. Walter Lowrie (Princeton, NJ: Princeton University Press) III, A, b, 1.

103 Ibid. III, A, a, 2.

104 Peter L. Berger and Thomas Luckmann, *The Social Construction of Reality* (Garden City: Doubleday, 1966) 94.

105 Becker, *Denial of Death*, 86–87.

106 Kierkegaard, "Sickness Unto Death," I, A. For Weber, Kierkegaard's compliant, servile self is one who adheres to the domination of "traditionalist authority." It refers to a psychic orientation to "the traditional workaday and to the belief in the everyday return as the inviolable norm of conduct." See "Social Psychology," 296.

107 Kierkegaard, "Sickness Unto Death," III, A, b. 2.

108 Becker, *Denial of Death*, 78.

109 Kierkegaard, "Sickness Unto Death," I, A.

110 Berger and Luckmann, *Social Construction of Reality*, 96.

111 Becker, *Denial of Death*, 75.

112 Kierkegaard, "Sickness Unto Death," III, B, 1, ii.

113 Becker, *Denial of Death*, 72.

114 Soren Kierkegaard, "Christian Discourse," in *The Essential Kierkegaard*, ed. Edward V. Hong and Edna H. Hong (Princeton: Princeton University Press, 1995) 312–332 at 324.

115 Kierkegaard, "Sickness Unto Death," II.

116 Wolfhart Pannenberg, *Anthropology in Theological Perspective*, trans. Matthew J. O'Connell (Philadelphia: Westminster, 1985) 58.

117 Max Scheler, *Man's Place in Nature*, trans. Hans Meyerhoff (Boston: Beacon, 1961) 91.

118 Kierkegaard, "Sickness Unto Death," III, A, b. 2.

119 Kierkegaard, "Fear and Trembling," in Lowrie, *Fear and Trembling and Sickness Unto Death*, Problemata: Preliminary Expectoration, 56, 57.

120 Ibid. 47.

121 Ibid. 48.

122 Ibid. Problem II, 90. Vico writes: "This brings us to the discovery of heroic virtue. For when human nature is of limited ideas and men have little capacity to understand the universal and eternal, they will be barbaric and ferocious, for these are indivisible properties of such a nature." See *The First New Science*, II, XXII, 137.

123 Becker, *Denial of Death*, 90.

124 Ibid. 29–30. Thomas Malthus, *An Essay on the Principle or Population and Other Writings* (London: Penguin, 2015) [orig. pub. 1798].

125 Sass, *Madness and Modernism*, 6.

126 Ibid. 14.

[127] Becker, *Denial of Death*, 63.

[128] Thomas Merton, "A Devout Mediation in Memory of Adolph Eichmann, in *Raids on the Unspeakable* (New York: New Directions, 1966) 46, 47.

Chapter 4

[1] Like the term used to describe them, the literary prophets, as opposed to prophetic figures such as Moses, Elijah, and Nathan are known for the books ascribed to them in the Hebrew Scriptures.

[2] Walter Brueggemann, *The Prophetic Imagination* (Philadelphia: Fortress, 1978) 9.

[3] Weber "Religious Rejections of the World," 328

[4] Weber, *Ancient Judaism*, 305.

[5] Harry Mowvley, *Reading the Old Testament Prophets Today* (Atlanta: John Knox, 1979) 21.

[6] Theodore E. Long, "Prophecy, Charisma, and Politics: Reinterpreting the Weberian Thesis," in *Prophetic Religions and Politics*, Vol. I, ed. Jeffrey K. Haddon and Anson Shupe (New York: Paragon, 1984) 3–17 at 3.

[7] Reid, *What Are They Saying about the Prophets?* 61.

[8] Ibid. 62.

[9] Mumia Abu-Jamal, *Death Blossoms* (Farmington: Plough Publishing, 1997) 1, 153.

[10] "The prophets are able to reproach us today quite as they reproached their contemporary Israel and Judah, and for precisely the same reasons ... We who share the prophets' faith do not read them aright if we are not sensible of the rebuke they offer continually to our complacency in the face of social and racial injustices, violations of the public trust, and other crimes that they condemned in the name of Israel's God and ours." Vawter, *The Conscience of Israel.*

[11] Rohr, *Everything Belongs*, 16.

[12] George Shulman, *American Prophecy* (Minneapolis: University of Minnesota Press, 2008) xiv.

[13] Ibid.

[14] Charlene Carruthers, "Hearing Assata Shakur's Call," *Women's Studies Quarterly* 46 (2018) 222–225 at 222.

[15] Ibid. 222, 224.

[16] Margo V. Perkins, *Autobiography as Activism* (Jackson: University of Mississippi Press, 2000) 1–2.

[17] Davis, *Angela Davis: An Autobiography*, xvi, 32.

[18] Perkins, *Autobiography as Activism*, 7.

[19] Kaveny, *Prophecy Without Contempt*, 44, 174.

[20] Orwell, *1984*, 255.

[21] Brueggemann, *The Prophetic Imagination*, 11.

[22] Crossley, *Jesus in an Age of Neoliberalism*, 41.

[23] Weber, *Ancient Judaism*, 314.

[24] Gerhard Von Rad, *The Message of the Prophets*, trans. D.M.G. Stalker (London: SCM Press, 1968) 38.

[25] Reid, *What Are They Saying about the Prophets?* 41. Harry Mowvley writes that there is "no evidence to suggest that the prophets ever set out to become prophets." Rather, the "prophet's response to this call is often one of disbelief, reluctance, and a feeling of inadequacy." See *Reading the Old Testament Prophets Today*, 19, 20.

[26] Von Rad, *Message*, 44.

[27] Abraham Heschel, *The Prophets* (New York: Harper & Row, 1955) 358.

[28] Weber, *Ancient Judaism*, 299.

[29] Heschel, *The Prophets*, 21.

30 Martin Buber, *The Prophetic Faith* (New York: Collier, 1949) 2–3, 244–245. Vawter takes a broader view of the *nabi*, asserting that the term is "ambiguous" in the Hebrew Bible. He notes that in I Sam 9: 9, the term is used to describe temple prophets who would, among other things, help someone locate a lost animal for a small fee. See *The Conscience of Israel*, 21.

31 Karl Rahner, *Theological Investigations Vol. XIII: Theology, Anthropology, Christology*, trans. David Bourke (New York: Crossroad, 1951) 167.

32 "The label sōpeh ('watchman,' 'sentinel') for the prophet was appropriate since the task of the sentinel posted on the city wall or the watchtower was to look out for danger approaching the city and warn those inside the walls in good time. The metaphor could therefore serve for the admonitory, and perhaps also the predictive role of the prophet in society." See Joseph Blenkinsopp, *Essays on Judaism in the Pre-Hellenistic Period* (Berlin: Gruyter, 2017) 18.

33 Ibid. 183.

34 Heschel, *The Prophets*, 18, 358.

35 Von Rad, *Message*, 20–21.

36 "The prophets were so free in taking over language for their own purposes that the precise nuances which they would have us catch in how they use a particular form are not easy to discern." Reid, *What Are They Saying about the Prophets?* 67.

37 Vawter, *The Conscience of Israel*, 6.

38 Von Rad, *Message*, 20–21.

39 Assata Shakur, *Assata: An Autobiography* (Westport: Lawrence Hill, 1987) 207.

40 Westermann, "God's Judgment and God's Mercy," 212.

41 Von Rad, *Message*, 33.

42 Westermann, "God's Judgment and God's Mercy," 212.

43 Martin Luther King, "Letter from Birmingham Jail," in *A Testament of Hope: Essential Writings and Speeches of Martin Luther King, Jr.*, ed. James Melvin Washington (San Francisco: Harper, 1991) 289–302 at 290.

44 Walzer, *In God's Shadow*, 104.

45 Shulman, *American Prophecy*, 5.

46 Von Rad, *Message*, 265–266.

47 Vawter, *The Conscience of Israel*, 213.

48 Weber, "Religious Rejections of the World," 337.

49 Ibid. 287–288. Concerning sin, Westermann writes: "The Old Testament knows no abstract and timeless concept of sin, which would be similar to a concept of being. Sins and transgressions are only mentioned when they threaten human existence, the human community, or the community between God and man." See "God's Judgment and God's Mercy," 213.

50 Heschel, *The Prophets*, 5.

51 Walzer, *In God's Shadow*, 107.

52 Shulman, *American Prophecy*, 5.

53 Ibid. 93–94.

54 Alexander Solzhenitsyn, *The Gulag Archipelago*, trans. Thomas P. Whitney (New York: Harper & Row, 1959) 25.

55 Ibid. 130.

56 Heschel, *The Prophets*, 9.

57 Camus' description of the "secular saint" mirrors mystical literature down through the ages as one who exercises "tremendous will power" and keeps "endless watch" on each breath, lest "in a careless moment" anything save "sympathy" be allowed to emit from the heart. See Albert Camus, *The Plague*, trans. Stuart Gilbert (New York: Knopf, 1993) 229–230.

58 Thomas Merton, "Rain and the Rhinoceros," in *Raids on the Unspeakable* (New York: New Directions, 1964) 9–23.

59 David Abram, *The Spell of the Sensuous* (New York: Vintage, 1996) 6.

60 George Jackson, *Soledad Brother: The Prison Letters of George Jackson* (New York: Bantam, 1970) 64.

61 Merton, "Rain and the Rhinoceros," 15.

62 Ibid. 18.

63 Kierkegaard, "Sickness Unto Death," III, B, b, 1, ii.

64 Heschel, *The Prophets*, 18.

65 Buber, *The Prophetic Faith*, 180.

66 Von Rad, *Message*, 18.

67 Ibid. 146.

68 Walzer, *In God's Shadow*, 74.

69 Schutt, *Homelessness and Housing*, 31.

70 Jens Soering, *The Convict Christ* (Maryknoll: Orbis, 2006) 18–21.

71 Heschel, *The Prophets*, 18.

72 Von Rad, *Message*, 74.

73 Ibid. 100.

74 Foucault, *Madness*, 58.

75 Victor Turner, *The Ritual Process* (Ithaca: Cornell University Press, 1969) 137.

76 Ibid. vii.

77 Ibid. 94.

78 Ryan Lee, *inter voice*, September 23, 2012, www.intervoiceonline.org/about-voices/personal-experience/share-your-story

79 Sass, *Madness and Modernism*, 14.

80 Neale and Oltmanns, *Schizophrenia*, 338.

81 Ibid. 289.

82 Laing, *The Politics of Experience*, 70.

83 Scull, *Social Disorder*, 328–329.

84 Heinz Cassirer, *Grace and Law: St. Paul, Kant, and the Hebrew Prophets* (Grand Rapids: Eerdmans, 1988) 94–95.

85 David Burrell speaks of the "exitus-reditus" theme, that all life comes and returns to God, as a dominant one in the Scriptures of the monotheistic religions. See *Toward a Jewish, Christian, Muslim Theology* (Chichester: Wiley Blackwell, 2011) 87, 96.

86 Cassirer, *Grace and Law*, 95.

87 Westermann, "God's Judgment and God's Mercy," 213.

88 Shulman, *American Prophecy*, 6.

89 Weber, "Religious Rejections of the World," 330.

90 Marilynne Robinson, *Gilead* (New York: Farrar, Strauss, and Giroux, 2004) 142.

91 Westermann, "God's Judgment and God's Mercy," 214.

92 Dubois continues: "We believe that at the bottom of organized human life there are necessary duties and services which no real human being ought to be compelled to do. We push below this mudsill the … half-men, whom we hate and despise, and seek to build above it—Democracy!" W.E.B. Dubois, "The Servant in the House," in *Darkwater: Voices from within the Veil* (New York: Harcourt, Brace, and Company, 1920).

93 Malcolm X, *The Autobiography of Malcolm X* (New York: Ballantine, 1965) 368–369.

94 Jackson, *Soledad Brother*, 62.

95 Skinner, *Beyond Freedom and Dignity*, 128.

96 Bernard J.F. Lonergan, *Insight* (New York: Philosophical Library, 1957) 179, 181. Kant says something similar: "To judge men in terms of their power of knowledge … we

divide them into those who must be granted *common sense* ... and men of *science*. Men of common sense are adept at dealing with rules as applied to instances; men of science at rules in themselves before they are applied. The understanding that belongs to the first type of power of knowledge is called *sound* human understanding; that belonging to the second type, an *acute mind*." Immanuel Kant, *Anthropology from a Pragmatic Point of View*, trans. Mary J. Gregor (The Hague: Martin Nijhoff, 1974) I, 6, 139 (italics in original).

97 Weber, "Social Psychology," 297.

98 Langer, *Philosophy in a New Key*, 266.

99 Bernard Lonergan, *Method in Theology* (New York: Herder and Herder, 1972) 238.

100 Ludwig Wittgenstein, *Philosophical Investigations*, trans. G.E. Anscombe (London: Basil Blackwell, 1098) 97.

101 Ibid. 101.

102 Wittgenstein, *On Certainty*, 356.

103 Schopenhauer, *The World as Will and Representation*, II, 29.

104 Alfred Schutz, *Collected Papers*, Vol. I, trans. Maurice Natanson (The Hague: Martinus Nijhoff, 1967) 227.

105 Ibid. 229.

106 Hegel, *Phenomenology of Spirit*, 69.

107 Grant Gillet, "Brain Pain," in *The Philosophy of Psychiatry*, ed. Jennifer Raddon (New York: Oxford University Press, 2004) 26. Erving Goffman states: "A social norm is that kind of guide for action which is supported by social sanctions, negative ones providing penalties for infraction, positive ones providing exemplary rewards for compliance. The significance of these rewards and penalties is not meant to lie in their intrinsic, substantive worth but in what they proclaim about the moral status of the actor." See *Relations in Public* (New York: Harper & Row, 1971) 95.

108 Kant, *Anthropology from a Pragmatic Point of View*, II, 67, 239–240.

109 Ibid. II, 69, 244.

110 Ibid. I, 24, 161.

111 Oliver Freudenreich, *Psychotic Disorders* (Philadelphia: Lippincott Williams & Wilkins, 2008) 4, 11.

112 Foucault, *Madness*, 115–116.

113 Williams, *Beyond Words*, 75, 91. I understand this to coincide, however, at least in part, with prophetic openness as Williams locates such linguistic innovation within a "context of grace" and a call for "renewal" that makes its recipients channels of divine "mercy."

114 Lonergan, *Insight*, 223.

115 Ibid. 191–193.

116 Ibid. 239.

117 Ibid. 228.

118 Ibid. 233.

119 Leo Strauss, *Early Writings*, trans. Michael Zank (Albany: State University of New York Press, 2002) 113.

120 Lonergan, *Insight*, 233.

121 Fingarette, *The Meaning of Criminal Insanity*, 77.

122 James, *Varieties*, Lecture 3.

123 Foucault, *Madness*, 101–102.

124 James, *Varieties*, Lectures 16–17.

125 Lonergan, *Insight*, 3–4.

126 Ibid. 193.

127 Ibid.

128 Wittgenstein, *Philosophical Investigations*, 500.

129 Ibid. 182.

130 Ibid. 130.

131 Whitehead, *Process and Reality*, 21.

132 Rieff, *Triumph of the Therapeutic*, 238–239.

133 Young, *The Exclusive Society*, 19.

134 Heschel, *The Prophets*, xvi.

135 Lonergan, *Insight*, 252.

136 Soering, *The Convict Christ*, 32–33.

137 Lonergan, *Insight*, 200.

138 Nussbaum, *The Fragility of Goodness*, 218.

139 Lonergan, *Insight*, 36.

140 Ibid. 4.

141 Langer, *Philosophy in a New Key*, 8.

142 Bey Z.K. Maakneru, "A Supreme Manifestation of Wisdom," 2016, *American Prison Writing Archive*, www.hamilton.edu/academics/centers/digital-humanities-initiative/projects/american-prison-writing-archive

143 James, *Varieties*, Lecture I.

144 Whitehead, *Process and Reality*, 4; Kant, *Critique of Pure Reason*, Introduction, VI, B, 21.

145 Jung, "Concept of the Collective Unconscious," 42–53.

146 Ulanov and Rosen, *Madness and Creativity*, 31.

147 Lonergan, *Insight*, 246.

148 Sass, *Madness and Modernism*, 25.

149 Schutz, *Collected Papers*, 123.

150 Edmund Husserl, *Ideas: General Introduction to Pure Phenomenology*, trans. W.R. Boyce Gibson (London: George Allen and Unwin, 1931) 12.

151 Ibid. 11–12.

152 Wittgenstein, *On Certainty*, 94, 105.

153 Lonergan, *Insight*, 47.

154 Ibid. 135.

155 Michael Arreygue, "Impetuous," October 15, 2016, *American Prison Writing Archive*, www.hamilton.edu/academics/centers/digital-humanities-initiative/projects/american-prison-writing-archive

156 Lonergan, *Insight*, 73.

157 Gillet, "Brain Pain," 33.

158 Lonergan, *Insight*, xi.

159 Cassirer, *Grace and Law*, 93–94.

160 Lonergan, *Insight*, 635.

161 Ibid. 514–515.

162 Ibid. 520

Chapter 5

1   Walter Brueggemann, *Tenacious Solidarity: Biblical Provocations on Race, Religion, Ecology, and Economy* (Minneapolis: Fortress, 2018) 384.

2   Mohamedou Ould Slahi, *Guantanamo Diary*, ed. Larry Sims (Boston: Back Bay, 2017) 216.

3   Ibid. 182.

4   Solzhenitsyn, *Gulag Archipelago*, 477.

5   Ibid. 147.

6   Ibid. 100–101.

7   Dubler and Lloyd, *Break Every Yoke*, 200. Slahi writes that at Guantanamo, "the war against the Islamic religion was more than obvious. Not only was there no sign to Mecca, but the ritual prayers were also forbidden. Possessing the Koran was also forbidden. Fasting was also forbidden. Practically any Islamic ritual was strictly forbidden." *Guantanamo Diary*, 261–262. Allison Liebling has written often about the necessity of penal environments to show fairness and respect toward the imprisoned in order to make their sentence "survivable." Where those basic human qualities are lacking, the psychological challenges experienced by captives can be both physically and mentally destructive. See, for example, "Moral Performance, Inhuman and Degrading Treatment and Prison Pain," *Punishment and Society* 13 (2011) 530–550.

8   Kenneth Hartman, "A Prisoner's Purpose," October 22, 2013, *American Prison Writing Archive*, www.hamilton.edu/academics/centers/digital-humanities-initiative/projects/american-prison-writing-archive

9   De Young, *Madness*, 24.

10   Otto, *The Idea of the Holy*, 177–178.

11   Nobody, "Reflections from the Cement Coffin," July 12, 2013, *American Prison Writing Archive*, www.hamilton.edu/academics/centers/digital-humanities-initiative/projects/american-prison-writing-archive

12   Laing, *The Politics of Experience*, 93. St. Augustine, *Confessions*, trans. R.S. Pine-Coffin (London: Penguin, 1961) Bk. XI.

13   Heidegger, *Being and Time*, 180.

14   Jaspers, *General Psychopathology*, 763.

15   Kierkegaard, "Sickness Unto Death," II.

16   Becker, *Denial of Death*, 63.

17   Otto, *The Idea of the Holy*, 22.

18   L. Mack-Lemdon, "Aramark food corporation scandal," July 5, 2018, *American Prison Writing Archive*, www.hamilton.edu/academics/centers/digital-humanities-initiative/projects/american-prison-writing-archive

19   Fisher et al, "Beyond Criminalization," 553.

20   St. John Climacus, *The Ladder of Divine Ascent*, trans. Archimandrite Lazarus Moore (New York: Harper & Brothers, 1959) Step 5, 10.

21   James Gilligan, *Preventing Violence* (New York: Thames & Hudson, 2001) 38.

22   Louis Dumont, *Homo Hierarchicus*, trans. Mark Sainsbury, Louis Dumont, and Basis Gulati (Chicago: University of Chicago Press, 1966).

23   Gilligan, *Preventing Violence*, 37, 44.

24   Ibid. 118.

25   Ibid. 119.

26   Ibid. 118.

27   Barbara Harlow, *Barred Women: Writing and Political Detention* (Hanover: Wesleyan University Press, 1992) 11.

28   Weber, "Social Psychology," 300.

29   Reginald Dwayne Betts, "House of Unending," in *Felon* (New York: W.W. Norton, 2019) 83.

30   Kierkegaard, "Christian Discourses," 314.

31   Fisher et al, "Beyond Criminalization," 549–550.

32   Hans Urs von Balthasar, *A Theological Anthropology* (New York: Sheed and Ward, 1968) 101.

33   T.J. Gorringe, *A Theology of the Built Environment* (Cambridge: Cambridge University Press, 2002) 82.

[34] Feeley and Simon, "The New Penology"; Loic Wacquant, "Probing the Meta-Prison," in *The Globalization of Supermax Prisons*, ed. Jeffrey Ian Ross (New Brunswick: Rutgers University Press, 2013) x.

[35] Kermet Reiter, *23/7: Pelican Bay Prison and the Rise of Long-Term Solitary Confinement* (New Haven and London: Yale University Press, 2016) 7.

[36] Harlow, *Barred Women*, 19.

[37] Ibid. 10.

[38] Leena Kurki and Norval Morris, "The Purposes, Practices, and Problems of Supermax Prions," *Crime and Justice* 28 (2001) 385–424 at 388.

[39] Abu-Jamal, *Death Blossoms*, 143–144.

[40] Roy D. King, "The Rise of the Supermax," *Punishment and Society* 12 (1999) 163–186 at 167.

[41] Reiter, *23/7*, 2–3.

[42] Laurna A. Rhodes, "Supermax as a Technology of Punishment," *Social Research* 74 (2007) 547–566 at 551.

[43] Wacquant, "Probing the Meta-Prison," xiii.

[44] King, "Rise of the Supermax," 171.

[45] Kurki and Morris, "Purposes, Practices," 388–389. See also Reiter, *23/7*, 2–3.

[46] Ibib. 421.

[47] Ibid. David Garland is among the many criminologists who point to the power of public opinion to shape correctional policy, however ill-founded may be the assumptions upon which that policy is based: "There is a new and distinctly populist current in penal politics that denigrates expert and professional elites." These fear-driven movements "begin with a much darker vision of the human condition. They assume that individuals will be strongly attracted to … antisocial and criminal conduct unless inhibited from doing so by robust and effective controls." See *The Culture of Control* (Chicago: University of Chicago Press, 2001) 13, 15. See also, Julian V. Roberts, Loretta J. Stalans, and David Indemauer, *Penal Populism and Public Opinion: Lessons From Five Countries* (New York: Oxford University Press, 2002); Michael Tonry, "Rebalancing the Criminal Justice System in Favour of the Victim: The Costly Consequence of Populist Rhetoric," in *Hearing the Victim: Adversarial Justice, Crime Victims and the State*, ed. Anthony Bottoms and Julian V. Roberts (Uffcolme: Willan Publishing, 2010) 72–103; Samuel Walker, *Popular Justice* (New York: Oxford University Press, 1980) 3.

[48] Kurki and Morris, "Purposes, Practices," 421.

[49] Lisa Guenther, "Subjects without a World: A Husserlian Analysis of Solitary Confinement," *Human Studies* 34 (2011) 257–276 at 265. Kurki and Morris write: "We have no doubt that supermaxes regularly hold psychotic and seriously mentally ill prisoners … many … are getting worse … and more psychologically disturbed." See "Purposes, Practices," 421.

[50] Rhodes, "Supermax as a Technology of Punishment," 548. See also Alex Vitale, "The School to Pipeline" in *The End of Policing*.

[51] Rhodes, "Supermax as a Technology of Punishment," 552. See also Jonathan Simon, *Governing Through Crime* (New York: Oxford University Press, 2007).

Conclusion

[1] Brenner, *Mental Illness and the Economy*, 4.

[2] Karl Polanyi writes: "To separate labor from other activities of life and to subject it to the laws of the market was to annihilate all organic forms of existence and to replace them by a different type of organization, an atomistic and individualistic one … To represent this principle as non-interference, as economic liberals are wont to do, was merely the

expression of an ingrained prejudice in favor of a different kind of interference, namely, such as would destroy non-contractual relations between individuals and prevent their spontaneous re-formation." See *The Great Transformation*, 163.

3   Brenner, *Mental Illness and the Economy*, 6.

4   Lofland, *Deviance and Identity*, 302.

5   Emil Brunner, *Man In Revolt*, trans. Olive Wyon (Philadelphia: Westminster, 1947) 29.

6   Kierkegaard, "Sickness Unto Death," III, b, 1.

7   Georg Wilhelm Friedrich Hegel, *Lectures on the Philosophy of Religion, Vol. 1*, trans. R.F. Brown, P.C. Hodgson, and J.M. Stewart (Berkeley: University of California Press, 1984) 102.

8   Ibid. 89, 105.

9   Sartre, *Being and Nothingness*, I, I, V.

10   Lacan, *Speech and Language in Psychoanalysis*, 9, 32.

11   Luhrmann, *Of Two Minds*, 44–45.

12   Luigi Pirandello, *One, No One, and One Hundred Thousand*, trans. William Weaver (Sacramento: Spurl, 2018) 118 [orig. pub. 1926].

13   Jaspers, *General Psychopathology*, 21.

14   Foucault, *Madness*, 192. Porter adds that "it is important to get inside the heads of the mad. For one thing, their thought-worlds throw down a challenge, being at once so alien and yet so uncannily familiar, like surrealist parodies of normality. For another, if we are to understand the treatment of the mad, we must not only listen to the pillars of society, judges and psychiatrists: their charges must be allowed a right of reply." See *Madmen*, 229–230.

15   Brunner, *Man In Revolt*, 18.

16   William R. Miller and Stephen Rollnick, SJ, *Motivational Interviewing* (New York and London: Guilford, 2002) 4, 5, 9.

17   Pascal, *Pensees*, trans. W.F. Trotter (New York: The Modern Library, 1941) 441 [orig. pub. 1670].

18   Brunner, *Man In Revolt*, 45.

19   Kierkegaard, *Fear and Trembling*, Problem II.

20   Kierkegaard, "Christian Discourses," 314.

21   Becker, *Denial of Death*, 200.

22   Rieff, *Triumph of the Therapeutic*, 35.

23   John Lofland and Rodney Stark, "Becoming a World Saver: A Theory of Conversion to a Deviant Perspective," *American Sociological Review* 30 (1965) 862–875 at 871.

24   Brunner, *Man In Revolt*, 9.

25   Reinhold Niebuhr, *Moral Man Immoral Society* (New York: Charles Scribner's Sons, 1932).

26   Webb, *Toward a Theology*, 129.

27   Plato, "Phaedrus," 106.

28   Ibid. 107.

29   Plato, "Phaedo" in *Plato: Six Great Dialogues*, 35–92 at 62.

30   Friedrich Nietzsche, "The Birth of Tragedy," in *The Birth of Tragedy and the Genealogy of Morals*, trans. Francis Gollfing (Garden City: Doubleday, 1956) I, iv.

31   Foucault, *Madness*, 80–81.

Index

References to endnotes show both the
page number and the note number (145n39).